Wellness
1 2 3

Simple Steps to
a Healthier, Younger You

Dr. Michael Koschade

Wellness 1 2 3

ISBN-13: 978-0-9988546-1-8
ISBN-10: 0-9988546-1-1

Published by: Celebrity Expert Author
http://celebrityexpertauthor.com

Canadian Address:
1108 - 1155 The High
Street,
Coquitlam, BC, Canada
V3B.7W4
Phone: (604) 941-3041
Fax: (604) 944-7993

US Address:
1300 Boblett Street
Unit A-218
Blaine, WA 98230
Phone: (866) 492-6623
Fax: (250) 493-6603

Table of Contents

Table of Contents

Introduction

"...your health IS everything and without it you have nothing. When you understand the basics, you can regain, rebuild and create health freedom for you and your family"

Getting through life happy and healthy can be a struggle...a real struggle. For many of us staying healthy or regaining our health can be one of the biggest challenges and mysteries. All of us have realized at some point that our health affects everything we do and everyone we know.

Some time after our "superstar and idealistic" 20s end, our 30s and 40s follow far too quickly...and life gets serious! The superstar loses some of the sparkle and shine, and idealism gets replaced with trying to simply "be happy" and accept things as they are.

It starts creeping up on us, slowly, in the mirror, on our waistlines, in our joints, on our face, and in our smile. The ease with which we used to glide through life now feels like it constantly needs some WD40. The energy, eagerness, and the confidence we once had are silently replaced. One by one, we slowly give up some of our hobbies, favorite sports, and pastimes. In the back of our minds, we live

with false, age- old mantras that get passed down from father to son, mother to daughter, from the six o'clock news,
radio reports, internet "experts", advertising campaigns,
and the many very believable myths. They all tell us the
same thing: getting old, sick, sore, and tired, is just a *normal* part of aging, and there's not much you can do about
it. Right? Isn't that what most people believe to be true?

    It may be what most people think, but it's not true, and
I'm here to tell you the "why" and the "how."

    The reality is that your health IS everything, and with-
out it, you have nothing. Statistically speaking, most of
us *can* and *will* face some pretty big health hurdles in our
lives. Sadly, too many of us falsely think that the statistics
mean "*luck of the draw,*" and so we keep our fingers crossed
and hope that bad things won't happen to us. Most of us
have never learned how easy it is to stay healthy and vibrant, or regain our health after a bout of illness. Without
learning a few simple secrets and understanding the simplicity and power that heals your body, far too many of us
end up cutting our lives short. We shrink our lives down
unnecessarily thinking this is how nature intended it to be.

    Wouldn't it be nice if taking control of your health were
really easy and if once and for all, you could understand the
"how" and the "why" of health and disease? You might be
surprised at how simple it is! The majority of people never
learn this and waste years riding the health and illness roll-
ercoaster...mostly coasting downhill.

    The good news is that it is really easy to regain, protect,
and enhance your health! That's what this book is all about.
There is a way to cut through all the misconceptions and
the overload of inaccurate information about health. There
are only a few important basics you need to know and a

couple of secrets that will jump-start your healing and health, bringing back your energy and vitality, naturally!

I've been studying, teaching and practicing healthcare and the lifestyle sciences for over 20 years, and feel fortunate to be able to say that I absolutely love what I do each day. As much as it's been fantastically rewarding to help thousands of patients and clients, along the way I also became my own working laboratory. I have gone through enough debilitating back pains, various joint problems in the knees, shoulders and wrists, skin problems, serious inflammatory conditions, extreme allergies and neurological changes from accidental toxic chemical exposure.

None of these experiences was fun, and some were downright scary. But, they all forced me to learn and figure out how to heal and become stronger, even though the calendar was telling me that I was getting older.

I am here to tell you that you CAN reverse the calendar. You can regain your energy, vitality, and the spring in your step. Even if you think you never had it in the first place, you can get it now. You only have to learn how to go about it. You can strengthen your immune system, reduce sick days, prevent injuries, get back your mobility and your mojo, and beat the statistics! Yes, you will still be a statistic, but you'll be the "good news" statistics, like those 95-year-olds you hear about who are breaking world records in running, cycling, swimming or sky diving. You don't need to become a record-breaking athlete, but when you stay strong, vibrant, energetic, disease-free, and have lifelong independence, you will beat the stats and disprove all the myths. And the best part is that you get to live life on your own terms. It's called freedom. Health freedom.

So, let me tell you my story...

I became a chiropractor by first becoming a patient early on in life. At age 17 I got a factory job in Montreal, where we built very large solid wood doors for corporate office towers. From the raw wood to the finished and packaged product, loaded in a truck, we made hundreds of doors a week. This job consisted of gluing, planing, sanding, staining, varnishing, and finally packaging...all of which was done manually and required me to lift and flip these doors, that weighed more than me, hundreds of times a day! I did this job for several summers and during school breaks, and occasionally at other times too. I had a very strong work ethic and high quality standards, so they loved me. However, unbeknownst to me at the time, I was damaging my lumbar spine. That, along with lots of ski jumping in my teens and growing years, left me with a serious back pain crisis.

It got so bad that I could hardly drive a car or sleep through the night. On one family trip to Florida, the problem got worse and I ended up seeing a chiropractor for the first time. He did a very thorough exam, took x-rays, and gave me my first adjustment.

Still not knowing what I wanted to do in life, I asked him how long it takes to become a chiropractor. When he told me "eight years", I quietly said to myself, "forget that!"

The adjustment only helped a little and I never went back to see him during that vacation.

The pain came and went over the next few months, and when I finally had enough, my mom suggested I go see her chiropractor in Montreal, Dr. Christian Van Lierde. She had been seeing him for her migraine headaches for years and had great success.

Dr. Christian was the guy I needed to meet, because within three or four weeks, I was completely pain-free, and had more energy and better sleep than I had in a couple of years! It was then and there that I decided I wanted to become a chiropractor —however long it took. I wanted to do for other people what he did for me. I continued to go to see him even after the pain was gone because he explained to me that the healing process takes time and that the lack of pain did not mean my back was fully healed and strong again.

My fascination with the human body and how it works started way back in my first high school grade 7 biology class. Unlike many of my classmates, I loved biology and everything I was learning. Fast-forward to 11 years after high school, to January 1997, when I started to practice in a chiropractic wellness clinic north of Toronto. It took a couple of years into practice to realize how much I still had to learn!

I discovered that the health my patients and I took for granted in our 20s was not guaranteed in our 30s and 40s! I found out the hard way that I couldn't just "coast" anymore. After numerous health challenges of my own, spending lots of money on the wrong supplements, faulty and flawed science, the wrong therapies and sifting through all the misinformation about health, I gradually figured it out. And so the focus of my practice started to change from a pain-based practice, to a wellness and lifestyle practice. I knew that having a healthy spine and getting chiropractic adjustments could dramatically improve people's lives, but there was more to it. Getting back to basic sciences and biology, and understanding humans beings as part of nature, was the first step.

I am going to save you hundreds of thousands of dollars and 20 years of studying by sharing with you all you need to know about health and healing in my Understanding Health stories. And no science degree is required.

Sit back, enjoy, and find out how you can keep and improve your health for a lifetime.

Understanding Health Made Ridiculously Simple

To build a house, you first need a foundation. This story is the first step in building that foundation to help you break down the mysteries of health.

Puppy Love

Imagine you have a dog (Or maybe you do have one.) I am saying this because very often people take better care of their pets than they do of themselves. What are the basic and essential requirements to keep your dog healthy for the whole of his life? Well, there are three essentials, and you already know all of them. First of all, you will buy your dog the best quality food you know about, and can afford. If you have the choice between food that is highly processed, full of chemicals, fillers, artificial flavours and colours, or food that is clean and pure and made specifically for dogs, (and not for some other animal), then you will surely buy the latter version, every time. If you have the choice of giving your dog clean, pure water or polluted, chemically treated one, every single time, you will choose pure water. Secondly, you know that in order for your dog to be and stay healthy, you will need to take him for walks and play with him, every day.

Walk him, let him run, fetch a ball, wrestle, play, and have fun. Even though you are probably not a veterinarian or a scientist, you know that those things will keep him happy, active, and be good for his heart, lungs, muscles, bones, and brain. The third thing your dog needs is, love. He needs to get his hugs, his head scratches, belly rubs, and loving words of encouragement. You would not keep him in a cage, in a dark basement, and yell at him. Never. He needs to feel safe, feel loved, and feel like he's part of your life and part of your family.

These three essential ingredients (good nutrition, exercise, and love) are all equally important, and will keep your dog healthy and happy. If you do all that, you are not being an "extreme" dog owner, or following some new wave fad. You are simply following the laws of biology.

Not surprisingly, human being have the same basic needs.

That's the first block in our foundation. Stick with me and by the time you are done reading this book, you will be smarter than 95% of all average 40+ year olds! It isn't difficult, but it is critical to get it right so you don't waste your time, money, and energy.

Once you understand how to be healthy and stay healthy, there are three steps you need to take.

1. You need to know where you are. Find out where you score in your age group and see whether you are moving towards health or towards illness. There is a simple questionnaire you can fill out to see where you are. We can help you with that.

2. Identify your goals. What is most important to you? Where do you want to be? How do you want to feel and why do you want those things?

3. Choose which is the most efficient and works best for you.

Then, start reaping the benefits of having health freedom, knowing you are in control, and that you can live life on your own terms.

I have a second dog story...stay tuned, it will make you laugh.

Chapter 1:
The Top 5 Reasons
People Come to See Me

*"Pain is not the problem, pain is a signal your body sends to
your brain to let you know you have a problem."*

Would it surprise you if I told you that 8 out of 10 patients who walk through my door suffer from lower-back pain (which we commonly refer to as LBP)? Other common problems are neck pain, headaches, sciatica, as well as neck, shoulder, and arm pain.

If you have ever suffered from any of these conditions, you know how incapacitating they can be. If left untreated, they get progressively worse, to the point where you are in constant pain and discomfort. Fortunately, there are safe and effective ways to treat these kinds of afflictions. Let me explain how.

Problem # 1: Low Back Pain

When Mary, 38, came to my office, she complained that her lower back was hurting. Sometimes, she said, the pain was sharp and at other times dull and nagging. Because of this chronic discomfort, she couldn't sit, stand, or bend. Since Mary worked in an office, her job required her to sit at her desk for long periods of time and she found that she could no longer do that.

I am no stranger to lower back pain – if you recall, that was the reason for my first visit to a chiropractor at 17 – so I understood how it had impacted Mary's life.

In her case, sitting at her desk for hours each day had put tremendous strain on the lumbar spine.

There have been many studies done on the development and evolution of the human skeleton. The researchers found that we were never designed to sit in chairs, but, rather to stand, squat or lay down. So before the invention of the chair many centuries ago, humans used a lot of their core muscles on a regular basis and their backs were in a much better shape. Prolonged sitting, on the other hand, relaxes the core muscles, puts a downward pressure on the pelvis, and creates a lot of changes that aren't particularly healthy for the spine.

Also, we engage in a lot of activities that the human body was never designed for. Less than 100 years ago nobody did downhill skiing, or hockey, gymnastics, or any extreme sports that we now commonly engage in but which can disrupt the spine.

The way I helped Mary is pretty much the same way I work with other patients who complain of LBP.

First, I examine the spine quite thoroughly to determine which areas aren't moving as well as they should. And that's something that chiropractors become very, very good at, because our hands can "read" the spine, so to speak; we can read it the way a blind person reads Braille.

Over time, we train our fingertips to become very sensitive, and we can determine which areas of the spine don't move as well as other areas. And sometimes, with feedback from the patient, we can tell if there is pain or tenderness. Once I find those areas, I adjust that part of the spine so that it starts to regain proper motion and function. For comparison purposes, I'll make note of each vertebra that isn't moving properly and, or is painful. That way when I'm doing a progress exam I can measure the exact results.

Finding those areas of reduced motion in the spine is a specific skill that only chiropractors have, that takes years of experience to develop

After a few weeks of regular adjustments, Mary's lower back pain disappeared. What was important in her case was to identify which of her habits are that cause the LBP, and to give her strategies to improve those habits. Getting rid of the pain without knowing what caused it, is only dealing with half the problem.

Problem #2: Neck Pain

Like LBP, neck pain is very common. Just think: on average, an adult human head weighs approximately 13 pounds, so day in and day out, our neck carries the weight equivalent to a large bowling ball!

That heavy weight is on top of the cervical spine, that is, the neck. And since we spend so much of our time sitting, our posture changes to what we call a "forward head posture" - sticking forward out of alignment from our shoulders. This puts a lot of strain on the neck. And that 13 pounds suddenly feels as heavy as 40 or 50 pounds, because it's not sitting straight on top of the spine anymore; it's leaning forward.

This was the case with a patient of mine named George who suffered from tremendous neck pain. Like so many other people I treat in my practice, he lost the ability to turn his head all the way to his shoulder. George was in his early 40s, but I've seen people of all ages who had lost their range of motion in the neck, so this problem is very common. And when you start to lose the full range of motion in your cervical spine, or any part of your spine, that's premature aging.

It's a gradual process. We can lose several degrees over a couple of years and not notice it because if our head doesn't turn as far as it used to, we compensate with our upper body. We'll turn our shoulders, and we don't even realize that we've started to lose some of our normal range of motion.

When someone like George comes to me, I want see where their restrictions are, and using my hands and fingertips I'll check all the vertebrae in the spine. There are only seven vertebrae in the neck, but I check how they're moving on the right and left side, and determine where those misalignments or blockages are. The scientific term for this condition is subluxation. Subluxations are kind of like the "rusty" joints in your spine.

I'll also examine the rest of the spine, especially the upper back, between the shoulder blades, as this area can have a contributing effect on the tension in the neck.

The loss of George being able to turn his neck properly, and without pain, was really affecting his day to day life. He was having trouble checking his blind-spot while driving. He was in pain working at his desk job. He was not able to concentrate and it was making him more and more irritable and short tempered. He told me it was getting in the way of his real, happy, personality.

George felt much better after I adjusted him and gave him specific exercises he can do at home and at the office. We discovered that his daily commute in the car and the many hours of computer work had also locked up his upper back, and so we worked together on improving his whole spine and general posture.

There are simple, yet very important "ingredients", so to speak, to getting your spine to stay healthy and mobile for your whole life, and when you learn them, you can greatly restore or improve your mobility and effectively "reverse the clock".

When I have exact measurements and have made notes on your whole spine I can easily compare and quantify your improvements. You'll see the numbers improve, and you'll also notice how great your spine starts to feel overall.

Over the years I've seen this in so many patients. Like George, when neck mobility is restored and tension is decreased, people feel younger and happier.

Problem #3: Headaches

There are different types and forms of headaches, but the most common are the tension-type stress headaches. Many of them are caused by misalignments in the neck, right at the base of the skull. When you run your fingers along the bottom of your skull and go just below the bony ridge, that's where your first cervical vertebrae lies, which we call C1. Along with C2, the second cervical vertebrae, it is where the most common misalignments, or subluxations, related to headaches occur.

The good news is that even people who suffer from chronic headaches for years can find relief with chiropractic treatment. I remember a 16-year-old patient who had a headache every day for one year straight. Imagine how distraught that girl was when she came to see me. Fortunately, after her first adjustment, her headache disappeared and never returned. She was so happy to get her life back. Her stomach, liver and kidneys were happy too not to have to deal with daily pain meds.

We continued to adjust for a few weeks, gradually decreasing the frequency of her adjustments, just to make sure the headaches didn't return.

We can never assume that the pain – be it headache, LBP, or any other ailment – will be gone with one adjustment. More often than not, a series of treatments are needed. But in this girl's case, since she was so young, healthy, and flexible, her headaches disappeared with one adjustment.

This happened early on in my career, before everyone was texting and spending so much time with their heads bent forward, looking down at a phone. I have since noticed an increased trend of young people with headaches, neck and upper back pain.

Now, what about migraines? They are more severe than tension headaches. Migraines are often accompanied by other symptoms like nausea, visual disturbances, and light sensitivity. While tension headaches frequently strike in the back of the head, on the temples, or above the eyes, migraines will typically present themselves on the same side of the head.

The treatment for migraines is pretty much the same as for tension headaches. I adjust the patient and, because I'm lifestyle-based, I'll look at what their nutrition and exercise status is, and where it can be changed and improved in order to prevent further incidents.

Problem #4: Sciatica

A while ago, a new patient, Justin, limped into my office and said, "Help me doctor, I've been diagnosed with sciatica."

Actually, "sciatica" is not a diagnosis on its own, but I knew what Justin meant. It's a pain down the leg, which can present itself in a few different patterns; the most common one is where it goes from the lower back or the buttocks down the back or the side of the leg.

The sciatic nerve is the largest nerve in the leg. It originates from the lumbar spine and sacrum, and goes down through the thigh. At the knee, it branches out into two nerves - kind of like a fork in the road. So the pain can present itself in the side and the back of the thigh, or go around into the groin, down below the knee, and even into the foot, heel, and toes. So any combination or any variation of that can be called sciatica, because those are all branches off the sciatic nerve.

Justin complained of severe pain shooting down his thigh. After examining him, I found that the problem came from his lumbar spine. In most cases, the lumbar spine or the pelvis are the major causes of sciatica.

If the cause is lumbar spine, I adjust it the same way I would for the lower back pain. In the pelvis, there is a small muscle called "piriformis," which rotates the leg. The sciatic nerve runs very close to it and when the piriformis muscle is very tense or tight, it can put pressure on the sciatic nerve. This can cause several different reactions: a lot of pain, or a loss of sensation, a "pins and needles" sensation, or a weakness in the leg muscles. The most common combination I find is pain down the back of the thigh and weakness in one of the hip flexor muscles.

During the examination and before the adjustment, I always check the patient's leg muscles and compare left and right muscle strength. I'll often find a weakness in the one or several of the muscles, typically on one side only. And that's one of the things I love showing people when I do the first adjustment and then test it again immediately afterwards. It's amazing for the patient to see how much of the power and the strength in that leg can come back with one adjustment. It doesn't mean that the whole problem is solved right there and then, but Justin was pleasantly surprised to see the correlation between adjusting his spine and how much strength returned in his leg, and how much better he felt afterwards.

Problem #5: Neck, Shoulder, and Arm

This kind of pain can start in the lower part of the neck or upper back area, almost always off to one side. The pain can shoot down into the shoulder itself, into the front of the shoulder and the chest area, or collarbone area. It could also spread between the shoulder blades and go right down the arm toward the elbow. Sometimes it even affects the hand and the fingers, and will have a similar presentation to the sciatica - pain or numbness and tingling, or a feeling of a weakness.

A patient of mine is an auto mechanic and has had a problem holding his tools, because his dominant hand and arm became very weak. I have a machine that can check patient's grip strength, and I can compare right to left and to what's normal. I determined that this particular patient had a subluxation, or a blockage, in his lower neck, which I then corrected with adjustments. The power came back to his hand before he even walked out of the room.

This is what I usually do with the neck, shoulder, and arm pain: I look at where exactly the subluxations are, and then use specific chiropractic adjustments to restore proper motion and remove any pressure exerted on that nerve, so that the nerve can flow properly again and bring strength back to those muscles.

A Multitude of Benefits

These are the top 5 reasons people come to see me, but I often treat other conditions as well. For instance, I have patients with digestive issues such as constipation, and once I adjust certain areas in their mid-back, it totally changes their digestive patterns and can help them restore it back to normal. And just recently I had a patient who complained of constant buzzing in her right ear. When I examined her neck and checked for the subluxation, she said, "Oh, it's already gone." But I did a full adjustment and yes, the buzzing did disappear.

Another common concern people come to see me with is a sudden onset of rib pain, or a sharp pain on one side between the shoulder blades. In some cases it can be quite severe and really scare people. Very often the pain is made worse with coughing, sneezing or laughing.

Why would this be a chiropractic issue, you may ask? Well, the spine between your shoulder blades, your upper back, has joints connecting each rib. It is so common for the upper back to be highly tense these days, and so these joints can get irritated and stuck. There are many reasons why this may suddenly happen, which we can discover by taking a thorough history and examining the spine. Adjusting the upper back and teaching proper posture exercises is the easiest and quickest remedy for this. I have had people who could hardly breathe because it was so painful and with a few adjustments they could start to get back to normal. In order for this not to return in the future we have to address the root cause. This usually involves some chiropractic corrective care and easy home spinal motion exercises.

There are also other, direct and indirect, benefits of chiropractic treatments. For instance, I hear patients complain of insomnia or generalized poor sleep. But after being adjusted, the most common feedback I get from them is that they sleep much better. That's because there is less pain and tension in their spine. And getting a restful night's sleep gives us more energy and, in turn, makes us happier. So patients come in to relieve their pain but get many more positive side effects from getting adjusted!

You might be wondering whether one chiropractic adjustment is sufficient to resolve a patient's problem. It can happen, but in most cases a series of treatments is recommended.

Generally, people come to me with pre-existing conditions, so full treatment requires several visits. It's true that just one adjustment can bring relief, but if the treatment is not continued, the underlying problem will not be properly corrected and it will resurface in the future. So the typical pattern is roughly three times a week for approximately four weeks, and then, depending on how much progress the patient has made, we may stay at that frequency or we may start to reduce it and put more time between the adjustments.

This timeline is not just based on my own experience, but also on scientific research. It shows that in people who stop right after the initial treatment, the pain that had brought them to a chiropractor in the first place re-emerges, and they are back to the way they were. However, those who have follow-up adjustments every two weeks will continue to improve, or at least maintain the improvement that they had.

Points To Remember:

All the examples outlined above show that pain and discomfort in various parts of your body can be relieved or eliminated with regular chiropractic treatment. As incapacitating as lower back pain, neck pain, headache, sciatica pain, and arm, shoulder, and neck pain are, there *is* effective treatment for all these – and many more – conditions.

In the next chapter, I'll talk about a very important topic – the real results and benefits you can get with chiropractic treatment. Stay tuned!

Chapter 2:
The Results and Benefits
You Can Get

*"Progress is what happens when you take a small baby step
and then you take two"*
-Dr. Mike

"See it big, keep it simple"
-Wilferd Peterson

In the previous chapter I talked about how chiropractic care can alleviate pain in the lower back, neck, head, arms, shoulders, as well as shooting pain caused by sciatica.

Pain relief is just one aspect of my practice. There are many more benefits that come from regular chiropractic adjustments and lifestyle care. Let's have a look.

Benefit #1: Increased Mobility and Flexibility

As I tell my patients. "You are only as young as the flexibility of your spine and your mind." I find this to be true because both spinal and mental mobility are incredibly important, especially as we age. Why? Because good flexibility helps prevent injuries, decreases pain, helps us sleep more comfortably, and helps us move through our normal daily activities with greater ease. A flexible mind allows us to embrace new ideas, be open to new possibilities, learn new things, and when we are learning, we are growing as individuals.

How many times have you heard people say they "strained" or "sprained" or otherwise hurt various parts of their body because they made a "wrong" move or were doing something as simple as picking up a pen off the floor? Quite often, I bet! And we all know someone who dismissed a new idea only because they were too stubborn or "set in their old ways of thinking," even though that new idea would help them tremendously. Flexibility in your spine and your mind are the keys to flowing through life much easier, physically and mentally.

Have you ever seen elderly people walking all hunched over, stiff, rigid, and shuffling their feet? You know that they would have trouble bending over to pick up something off the floor or tying their own shoes. They very likely spend most of their time between different doctors' appointments and are on several different medications. Those are the kind of people who are more prone to injuries. Their quality of life is very low because it's directly correlated to their ability to move, bend, flex, reach, and twist. This loss of spinal motion affects quality of life; as people start to lose their normal range of motion, they start to do less. And the less we do, the more we shrink our lives. It becomes a vicious circle.

But then, you often see older people who are complete opposites of the stiff, hunched-over folks. They walk with straight backs and a good stride, swinging their arms. Those are the type of people who enjoy their senior years: They travel, play golf, and generally stay physically and mentally active. Very likely, they see their doctor only once a year for a check-up.

When I look at how someone moves, I can tell a lot about this person's overall health and quality of life. As a chiropractor, I certainly can see how people start to lose their mobility and flexibility in their spine. And very often, they start to lose it earlier than they realize. As I mentioned before, loss of range of motion is premature aging.

A while ago I had a patient, Joan. She was only in her early 50s, but was stiff all over and her joints hurt. She self-diagnosed her condition as arthritis. I treated her the same way I treat other patients with similar ailments – by adjusting her spine, addressing the inflammation in her joints. and by giving her spinal hygiene exercises. This restored her range of motion, flexibility, balance, and coordination.

There is actually scientific evidence to support this. Some years ago, researchers at University of Melbourne in Australia performed a study using 105 patients who complained of stiffness and loss of flexibility. There were three groups in this study: In one, participants were not treated at all; in the second, they were given "fake" adjustments; and in the last one they received "real" chiropractic adjustments. Those who received the proper chiropractic care showed a considerable increase in their range of motion, while the others did not.

So, as you can see, chiropractic adjustments are beneficial in improving flexibility and range of motion, while reducing stiffness and pain.

Benefit # 2: Prevent and Reverse Joint Conditions and Arthritis, Reduce Pain and Inflammation

So many people – including my patient Joan I mentioned above – tell me: " Doc, I'm getting old and I'm in constant pain. It must be arthritis." People just naturally assume that arthritis is inevitable in middle age and up.

But not all inflammation is considered bad or can be blamed on arthritis. If you twist an ankle or damage a knee, sometimes they swell up, and you can see from the outside that there's some inflammation in there. This is considered a normal part of the body's healing process, it is necessary and important. But when you have inflammatory body chemistry due to nutritional deficiencies or toxins, and it's all throughout your body, you may not even realize this is happening and just think your knuckles or other joints ache because you're getting old or have arthritis, or that it's normal for your age to feel this way.

People tend to turn to medications to relieve their pain and reduce swelling, but other than that, they continue the same lifestyle as before, which likely caused the inflammation in the first place. But there is a simpler and healthier way to tackle this problem: by changing the diet and adding things that we're deficient in, we can make some really big changes.

Years ago, I occasionally filled in for another chiropractor, Dr. Ken Dick. I'd been studying Omega-3s for so many years and it's always on top of mind. One day a patient came in. She was around 70 years old and 25 years earlier she had been diagnosed with rheumatoid arthritis, which is considered an autoimmune disease.

She was put on some anti-inflammatory and immune suppressing medications, which have horrible side effects.

I gave her information on Omega-3 and directed her to a high-quality brand that she could purchase and start taking right away. And then, because she wasn't my patient, I didn't see her again until the following year when I was filling in for the same chiropractor. She told me that within approximately six weeks of starting the Omega-3 supplements, she was feeling so much better that she was reducing a whole bunch of her medications she'd been taking for years.

She told her friends who had also been diagnosed with rheumatoid arthritis, about the importance of Omega 3s. After they started taking it, they too saw their inflammation go down or disappear altogether.

How can this be, you may ask? Well, those of us living in western society are deficient in Omega-3s, specifically EPA and DHA. As we evolved over the millennia, we consumed a lot of Omega 3 fatty acids in the natural diet. It all came from the wild game and the animals that grazed on grass such as buffalo. People who lived near the sea received their required Omega 3s from the fish they ate. But as agriculture developed, farmers stopped feeding their cows grass. They switched to corn, which completely changed the meat, and it became very inflammatory. This meat is rich in Omega-6, which we require in equal amounts to Omega-3. So while we get plenty of Omega-6, we have become deficient in Omega-3. Some research suggests that we now have 24 or 25 times more Omega-6 than we require.

On the other hand, we severely lack Omega-3s, and that disproportionate ratio produces an inflammatory response in the body. And so many of modern-day illnesses are caused by inflammation. But the anti-inflammatory drugs that are so frequently prescribed can never replace what your body lacks. All they do is artificially reduce the inflammation, instead of correcting the root cause of the inflammation, which is why Omega-3 supplementation is so essential. It is not only essential for people with symptoms or diagnosed diseases, but for everyone because there are very few of us who eat the way our ancestors ate.

Our genetic code evolved and adapted to its environment over time with the regular and daily consumption of Omega 3 fatty acids, and it remains an <u>essential</u> requirement for cell function and health to this day. Research has shown that our genetic code is virtually unchanged in the last 20, 000 years. What has changed drastically is our food source and our lifestyle.

There were two reasons Dr. Ken's patient started to feel better after taking the Omega-3 supplements. One, her body finally received the essential nutrient it was sorely missing. And two, she was no longer exposed to the toxicity of all the drugs she had been taking for years.

I have seen this kind of dramatic improvement in many of my own patients as well.

Benefit # 3: Improved Neurological Response

All of the benefits listed above are inter-connected: Having a flexible spine has great implications on overall neurological function.

The spinal column is there to hold us up. It's a center core, a stability structure.

But its role is also to protect the spinal cord. And inside your spinal joints, there are millions of tiny sensors, which send nerve signals up into the back part of the brain, called the cerebellum. So when we have free-flowing non-stressed spinal joints that are moving in their natural state, they send up nerve signals to the brain. These are really important, healthy signals. And when the spine is restricted, when it is stuck, when those joints are inflamed and not moving, they send up a stress signal up to the cerebellum.

Motion is key. All movement and joint motion is important and healthy. But when you have proper *spinal motion*, your entire neurological system just works better, because motion of the spine runs the cerebellum; the cerebellum runs our cerebral cortex, which is the bigger, more advanced part of our brain.

The cerebral cortex, in turn, runs the ecosystem of the human body. Spinal motion is very important because the more flexible you are, the more coordinated your nervous system is. You have better balance and better stability, which are so crucial as we get older and are more prone to falls.

And, of course, there are all the mental benefits as well – if your brain function is optimal, you feel more alert and "with it." So many of today's mental and emotional problems are greatly improved by movement of the body. We are designed to move, work, walk and run. As more and more of us move less and sit more from young age on, we are noticing more and more mental and emotional disorders. Walking and exercising helps mood disorders and a great part of that is due to spinal motion stimulating the brain.

It may be hard to believe but I had a few patients who were yoga teachers and came to me for adjustments. Seems that even people as supple as yoga teachers can have restrictions in their spine and joints. It's part of our modern, sedentary lifestyle.

Whether my patients are yoga enthusiasts or not, I first identify areas that are restricted and / or inflamed. I then go through a series of adjustments to restore proper motion of the spine. The actual adjustment itself has quite a large neurological impact on the patient. There are all kinds of natural endorphins that are released, which are quite calming. This is why we often have people report that they slept better that day.

I also make sure the patients have their own nutritional program, and Omega-3 and vitamin D supplements are a part of that. I also give them some range-of-motion exercises so they can get their spine moving, which then also improves neurological function.

I already mentioned the importance of Omega-3, but what about vitamin D? One of the effects when we are deficient in vitamin D is increased inflammation. One of the benefits of increasing vitamin D, along with Omega-3, is to reduce inflammation. Unfortunately, those of us living in the Western or Northern Hemisphere don't have enough of this vitamin, which is created in our bodies through the exposure of UV-B light from the sun.

When humans moved away from the equator, we became more fair-skinned. We got a lot of our vitamin D through eating animal organ meats, as well as some of the fats, which is where many of the vitamins are stored. But because we don't eat like that anymore, and because our skin is almost always covered up, we get very little sunlight exposure. That's why most of us are very deficient in vitamin D.

Benefit #4: Weight Loss

As they age, many people start to put on extra pounds. Why we gain weight is not a mystery, it is simply that our lifestyle habits change. We become less active than we once were, giving up sports, getting outside, doing physical work, and we tend to sit more, drive more, walk less, and eat just as much or more food than we used to.

The body is genetically programmed to save those extra calories in the form of fat for times of famine. Our ancestors often came home from hunting empty handed. But how often have you come home to find no food in your house? If you are fortunate, never! Between ages 20 to 40, the average person gains 40 pounds. That's 2-pounds-per-year weight gain can easily go unnoticed as it's quite gradual.

Being overweight is not just an aesthetic problem - it can have quite an impact on the discs of your spine as well as on your knees, hip joints, and feet. In fact, whatever extra weight you are carrying is bad – not just for your back, knees, and joints, but also for your cardiovascular and respiratory systems, and overall health.

It is never too late (which means you are never too old) to try to lose weight and maintain the loss in a healthy way. It CAN be done.

I have a couple of rockstar patients, Francine and Dan, both in their 50s who each lost a tremendous amount of weight by following my weight loss program. It was and is life changing, on many, many levels.

Not too long ago, I had a patient in his early 40s, who weighed almost 500 pounds for most of his adult life. He had lost close to 300 pounds before coming to me but still had more weight to lose. At this young age, he had already had knee replacement surgery.

When I x-rayed him, his spine was one of the worst ones I've seen in 20 years of practice. It was so degenerated. There are certainly a lot of people carrying 100 pounds more than they should, though most are probably over-weight by maybe 20 to 50 pounds.

Like Francine and Dan, this patient too followed my medically developed program, which is based on a sensible weight loss protocol and emphasizes fat loss, while sup-porting and protecting one's muscle mass.

And while I am on the subject of weight loss, one of the other advantages of slimming down is having more energy. Everything you do throughout the day is just so much easi-er: Getting out of bed, walking up a flight of stairs, playing sports, or whatever else.

Once the extra pounds, as well as the pain and the strain on your spine, knees, and joints is gone, you can literally get your life back.

Benefit #5: Stress Reduction, Better Mood

In the beginning of this chapter, I talked about both physical and mental benefits of chiropractic treatment. I covered the physical aspects - like less pain, stiffness, dis-comfort, and tension – in the points above.

Actually, it's impossible to separate physical from men-tal. It's all connected. If you have a lot of stress in your life, it could manifest itself as a headache or another type of pain. And if any of your body parts hurt, it's difficult to be happy.

This is where a chiropractor can help. When Paul came to see me, he was very down emotionally. When I asked him why, he responded that his lower back hurt so much, he could no longer do the activities he used to enjoy and it was affecting his overall mood. Over the next several visits I adjusted Paul's spine, and also recommended Omega-3 and vitamin D supplements to reduce inflammation.

As he continues to come in for lifestyle care and maintenance adjustments, Paul reports that he has been experiencing less and less pain since he began his adjustments, and he has become more and more upbeat about his life. Finally getting back to doing the things he loves. When he had to give up some of his favourite sports and hobbies, it made him really unhappy. The domino effect that has in our lives is often underestimated.

That's how chiropractic adjustments and lifestyle care can improve our overall feeling and wellbeing.

Points to Remember:

As you can see, chiropractic adjustments and lifestyle care yield many advantages, such as increasing mobility and flexibility; reducing pain and joint inflammation; improving neurological response; helping to lose weight, and reducing stress. Anyone, regardless of age, can benefit from regular visits to a chiropractor, and feel happier and healthier.

In the next chapter, I will answer a question you may be asking yourself when visiting a chiropractor: "How did I get here and what will it take to get my results?"

It's a very pertinent question, so turn the page and read on!

Chapter 3:
How Did I Get Here, And What Will It Take To Get My Results?

"The only way to coast is downhill"
- Bill Esteb

In the next chapter, I'll explain what is involved in a chiropractic visit, from the time a patient comes in to when he or she leaves my office. For now, I will discuss the reasons that prompt my patients to come to me, as well as the transformation they see in their health and well-being after a series of visits.

Although the results may *seem* magical at times, I can assure you that there is nothing magical or mysterious about how the body regains and maintains health. It is all, no pun intended, hands-on!

Why do you need to see a chiropractor?

Before I answer this question, let me tell you about Thomas.

Not long ago, Thomas walked into my office. He didn't look happy at all. He said that he had tried all kinds of treatments and saw several doctors to help him with chronic neck pain. He was taking anti-inflammatory medications, which not only brought very limited relief, but also made him tired and not feel as well as he used to. He told me he had never been to a chiropractor before but was so desperate, he wanted to give it a try.

When I examined him, I discovered that, because of the pain and inflammation, he lost some of the normal range of motion in the neck. So after his examination was completed, I reviewed his X-rays and gave him a report of my findings. I adjusted him the same way I do all my patients who have this condition: I pinpointed areas where the misalignments and blockages were in his vertebrae and spine, and gave him very specific chiropractic adjustments to begin the correction of these misalignments. Thomas felt some relief immediately but I explained that, to improve upon and maintain those results, we needed to continue his adjustments to correct the problem so it doesn't recur. As part of my protocol, I also advised him to start taking Omega-3 and vitamin D supplements to address the inflammation. He followed my suggestions and, over several weeks, the flexibility and range of motion in his neck was restored, and the pain was gone.

Thomas is pretty typical of people I treat. Before patients come to see me, they have likely suffered from chronic pain in parts of their bodies – most commonly, as already covered in a previous chapter, lower back, neck, head, arms and shoulders, or sciatica pain.

Quite a few of them tried other treatments and medications, with little or no results. How do they end up in my office? Maybe someone they know recommended me to them, or perhaps, like Thomas, they decided to try a chiropractor as sort of a "last resort," hoping that, after so many failed attempts to find relief, a chiropractor will help them, at last.

Whatever reason brings patients to my office, I am happy to help them alleviate their pain and improve their quality of life.

The Holistic Approach

I already mentioned that my practice is lifestyle-based: It's not only about alleviating pain and simply masking the symptoms, but actually about *improving* overall health, making you stronger and better able to prevent the problem from recurring in the future.

So when patients come to see me, I take a look at the whole picture, so to speak. I don't just examine the body's structure—the spine—and how it functions (though that's certainly where I start and is a vital part of my examination).

Spine is very important, of course, but I also look at my patient's nutritional habits, thought patterns, physical activity, and other lifestyle factors that influence their physical and mental wellbeing.

After I have determined what their spinal problem is and what is needed to help restore it back to health, I give our patients a health-risk assessment (HRA) questionnaire. This covers the 3 main categories of health and wellness: physical habits, nutritional habits and emotional / thought patterns. Every one of the 65 questions in there is evidence-based, coming from the most current lifestyle sciences. For example, the questions will ask about how many hours a day you spend sitting. How many fruits and vegetables do you eat per day, and what level of happiness do you enjoy in your job. Along with 62 other detailed and specific questions, we can assess the strengths and weaknesses in your day-to-day habits.

This in-depth questionnaire gives me a good idea of the patient's habits and overall health. Once I've assessed where a person is on this "continuum of health" – or "wellness spectrum" – we can identify the areas that need improvement. This is intended to help make patients stronger and better able to resist relapses of their original complaint or illness in the future.

That's what the holistic approach is: Taking into consideration the complete person - physically, chemically (which includes nutrients, deficiencies and toxins), and emotionally (thought patterns and habits) - in order to improve health and prevent illness.

Getting the Results

Now that you know a bit about how I assess and work with my patients, -using an science-based, lifestyle approach, – you are probably wondering what it will take to get the results you want.

First thing you should know is that for any treatment or wellness protocol to be beneficial and complete, you, the patient, have to do your part and be actively involved in your recovery and future maintenance.

For instance, if you come to see me because of chronic back pain and you are carrying extra weight, it goes to reason that losing weight will be an important part of your future spinal care; the weight loss has to happen before you can be fully healthy and get better. Pain can disappear for a while, but that does not mean the spine is healthy.

Losing weight can be done in a number of ways and we have different options. For instance, you could be doing it on your own, meaning *self-guided*, using the HRA as your guide for what to change. Or you can choose to do a 90-day Lifestyle Plan that tells you everything you need to know about how to eat, exercise, and think for 90 days. This gives you a jump start on your recovery and is all supported by the most current lifestyle sciences! Another option is our one-on-one weight-loss coaching program used by many to get fast results in a healthy, monitored way. For any of these approaches *education is the key* to long lasting success. Knowing "how" and "why" is the most important part of improving your health and maintaining it for your entire life.

By having assessed various measurements, including range of motion, strength, posture, spinal misalignments (subluxations) and inflammation, we can track your progress together. You get to witness your overall improvements each time we do a progress exam. Because you are an active participant in this process, it makes it fun to watch your health scores improve. By assessing your overall health risks and habits, you can enjoy seeing yourself move closer to wellness and away from illness. It's quite an exciting and encouraging experience.

Depending on your personality, you may only want to change a few small habits at a time, or you may want to make a complete lifestyle change. The choice is always yours. The length of time it takes depends on a few variables such as your age, the length of time you have had a problem, and your willingness to address the necessary steps, pre-existing conditions, old unresolved traumas, or years of unhealthy habits.

Lifestyle habits are the greatest determining factors on where you are on the health spectrum. And the best part of that news is that with the right, scientifically based information we provide, you can be in control of your health.

But, if you want to see tangible, lasting results, you have to be patient. As I mentioned in Chapter 1, pre-existing, chronic conditions – be it back, neck, arms and shoulder, or sciatica pain – will not resolve themselves with just one single treatment. Full recovery – in other words, getting, and maintaining, the results you want – require a series of visits. This is even truer for an older person, since he or she has probably been struggling with the problem(s) for a long time.

Transformations

So far, I talked about a number of my patients who became pain-free and significantly improved their quality of life by getting regular adjustments, along with eating right, exercising, and taking Omega-3 and vitamin D supplements.

Another supplement I typically recommend is a good, non-dairy based probiotic. These supplements help build up and replenish the healthy bacteria inside your intestinal tract (also referred to as our Intestinal Flora). These healthy bacteria make up the largest portion of your immune system; some research suggests as much as 70-80% of your immune defense comes from these bacteria. This makes sense, since the digestive tract, from top to bottom, is your body's interface between the outside world and your inside world. This is where foods, nutrients, toxins, and any unwanted, potentially harmful organisms would come into contact with your insides, your blood stream, through absorption in the intestines. Having a large, strong army of soldiers waiting and ready at the border, completely makes sense, doesn't it? When those soldiers are strong and healthy and plentiful, they can take care of most, if not all, unwanted intruders.

Deficiencies of probiotic bacteria have been linked to greater risk of severe conditions/illnesses throughout life, including diarrhea, candida, digestive disorders, immune deficiency, allergies, asthma, eczema, dermatitis, vitamin deficiency, systemic infections, high cholesterol levels, cancers, heart disease, bladder infections, depression, and decreased overall health and vitality.

That's why it is important to take this supplement daily. Probiotics were once a normal part of our diet, yet we are almost all deficient nowadays due to the changes in agriculture and the many foods we consume that deplete or damage our natural intestinal flora.

Another patient of mine, Louise, came in for chiropractic care for her lower back, but when I reviewed her health questionnaire, I noticed that she complained of constant digestive problems. It turned out that she had previously been diagnosed with Irritable Bowel Syndrome (IBS), an inflammatory condition involving recurrent abdominal pain with diarrhea or constipation. I suggested that, along with Omega-3 and vitamin D to relieve inflammation in her back and the rest of her body, she also take a high quality brand of probiotics to improve her intestinal environment.

Louise started to feel the positive effect of these supplements within a few weeks, and she has continued with this regimen, along with regular adjustments of her spine. She is like a whole new person now!

Can you expect the same kind of transformation? Absolutely! But the progress you make depends only on you – on your commitment to getting healthy and sticking with the program.

Points to remember:

You can get great results from chiropractic care – for your spine, joints, and health in general - but you must be motivated to stay on course, be willing to change some of your previous habits, and adapt new ones. With the proper knowledge and guidance you can regain and maintain a level of health and wellbeing you desire.

Now that you know what it takes to get all the health benefits, let's look at what a typical chiropractic visit looks like.

Chapter 4:
What Does A Typical Chiropractic Visit Look Like?

*"Just as your dentist teaches you healthy dental
habits to protect your teeth and gums,
my role is to teach you what your spine needs
to stay strong and healthy
for your lifetime."*

If you have never been to a chiropractor, you may be wondering what to expect. So in this chapter I would like to take you, step by step, through a typical visit.

Some of the steps have already been explained in previous chapters but I will go through the process again, so it is all clear and holds no mysteries.

Okay, let's get started!

Step #1: Getting to Know The Patient

Before a patient climbs on the chiropractic table, we sit down and talk so that I can understand what brought him or her to me. Most people, as I already mentioned, complain of lower back pain – that's the most common condition I see. Many also suffer from neck, arms, shoulder, and sciatica pain. And a lot of people also need relief from tension headaches.

Although all these ailments are very common, the causes of the pain vary. For instance, Philip's chronic lower back pain resulted from carrying heavy loads of material at his job on a construction site, while Dana's back was hurting from constant and prolonged sitting at her computer. Yet another patient, David, suffered from both backache and sciatica pain because he was very overweight, and carrying those many extra pounds for years has put a lot of strain and pressure on his spine.

Another patient, Patrick, came to me complaining of dizziness. His medical doctor referred him to an ENT (Ear, Nose and Throat specialist), thinking that the dizziness was caused by disturbances in his inner ear. As it turned out, Patrick's ears were fine, but upon examination of his spine, I found he had a lot of tension in his neck and upper back, and discovered a misalignment of some of his cervical and thoracic vertebrae. This is not something that a medical doctor would likely consider, but a chiropractor does.

That's why it is very important to get to know the patient, how they spend their day, what kind of work, hobbies or sports they do, as well as his or her health history. This is also the reason why I rely on the health questionnaire I mentioned earlier. It lets me know not only what this particular person is suffering from now, but also what pre-existing conditions or injuries he or she sustained - not necessarily related to lower back pain or whatever other condition brought this individual to me, but other ailments as well. The more I know about my patient's health, the better I can help them.

The questionnaire is pretty thorough and comprehensive. Naturally, it asks about discomfort or pain in the spine, muscles and joints. But it goes much further than that. For example, it has questions relating to medications the patient may take; alcohol and tobacco use; nutrition and exercise habits; what position they sleep in; level of stress and irritability, and more.

Why is this questionnaire such a key component of the initial consultation? First of all, because it helps me get a good idea of the patients' habits, behavior, and health history. And secondly, because so many illnesses and conditions are interconnected; in other words, pain in various parts of the body don't just happen out of the blue, so it's important to know where it originates and why.

So the first step in the consultation is getting to know my patients very well.

Step #2: A Thorough Examination

Once I speak with the patient and get acquainted with the health history from the filled-out questionnaire, I proceed to examine and evaluate that person's condition.

My assistant and I will perform a spinal health assessment (more about it in a minute), checking the patient's functional abilities - how straight, strong, and flexible the spine is. We also check the range of motion, going vertebrae by vertebrae through the cervical spine, thoracic spine, and lumbar spine. We look for restrictions in the motion and to see if inflammation is present. So even if the patient complains of low back or neck pain, we always look at the whole spine.

Then, we score all the findings in a computer and complete the Spinal Health Assessment, or the SHA for short.

The SHA was developed by Dr. James Chestnut, and it allows us to accurately assess the patient's spinal health based on criteria such as mobility, strength, coordination, and other key factors. It is based on the latest research for spinal health and rehabilitation.

Some of the things I look at are the duration and frequency of symptoms, areas of pain and discomfort, and what makes the pain better or worse – for instance, sitting, moving, etc.

If necessary – and this is most of the time for adults, but rarely for children – I'll send the patients for X-rays. That will be usually done the same day. Before the end of the first visit, we'll book a second appointment during which we'll review the spinal health assessment and x-rays together.

As has been said, "a picture is worth a thousand words." Reviewing the X-rays together with the patient is a very interesting visual because, as a comparison, I show them X-rays of a perfectly healthy spine on a special chart, which also has a moderately and severely degenerated spine. This way, the patient has a good idea of where he or she falls on that spectrum.

At the same time, I will assess whether the patient needs orthotics, which are custom-made supports for the feet and arches. Fallen arches, flat feet and bunions can all have an impact on the knees, hips, lower back, and overall body alignment.

And because mine is a lifestyle-based practice, I may also do a body composition analysis, to determine the patient's level of risk for metabolic syndrome. This is to see how much body fat the patient is carrying in relation to height, weight, gender, and age group.

All these initial tests and assessments are typically done on the first visit or sometimes need to be finished on the second visit. On the second day, I review my findings with the patient and make a personalized care plan, as well as prescribe the exact dosage for the Omega-3, vitamin D, and probiotics.

At this time, I will also explain the importance of continued care. Sometimes people think that bodies just magically heal in a couple visits, so I make sure they understand the different phases of healing and the time it takes to see lasting results.

Research clearly shows that people who have continued care get much better results long term than those who come in just once or twice, or those who yo-yo and come in only once in a while when the mood – or the pain – strikes them.

The body needs to go through the three different healing phases properly to ensure that the problem doesn't return or become a chronic condition. The first two phases are a little shorter, and the last one is longer because the body is remodeling itself and all the tissues are becoming strong again. The three phases of healing are natural laws of biology and they cannot be skipped over. Similarly, there is an average healing and recovery time after common knee surgery. The healing process of the human body cannot be sped up any faster. After pain and symptoms have gone, the healing continues. This is a crucial time to continue supporting your initial care protocol. Time, exercise, rest, and proper nutrients are essential for any joint-muscle complex, be it your knee or your spine, so that they can heal properly and be strong enough to resume normal activity. Without going through the full three healing phases the areas never heal fully and you are prone to more easily re-injure the area.

Step #3: The Chiropractic Adjustment

First, I examine the spine quite thoroughly to determine which areas aren't moving as well as they should. I already mentioned that a chiropractor's hands can "read" the spine because over time our fingertips become very sensitive, helping us pinpoint the parts of the spine that don't move well.

And by the way, people of all ages – from newborns to seniors – can benefit from chiropractic adjustment, which I always tailor to each individual's size, age and particular health issue.

Recently, a patient asked me whether it is true that I will "crack" his bones when I adjust him. "Cracking" the bones is certainly a common way patients think about this procedure, but there is absolutely no "cracking" going on. When joint motion is being restored through chiropractic adjustments, there is a "release" of the joint pressure, and that creates a "popping" sound. There are several ways to adjust the spine. Sometimes I will use light pressure, at other times an adjusting instrument is used, and most commonly I manually apply a very quick, specific thrust to the affected joint and a popping sound – not a crack – can be heard.

Many patients also wonder if an adjustment is painful. I will answer many of the most common questions I get in the last chapter of this book, but for now I can assure you that the typical adjustments themselves do not hurt (if they did, people would not come back for multiple visits!)

Sometimes patients are in acute pain when they arrive and the area is inflamed and sensitive, so anyone touching the area will induce some pain. We are trained to minimize the discomfort of our patients and recommend measures to help create comfort as quickly as possible.

As a matter of fact, the overwhelming majority of my patients report a sense of well-being and ease after their adjustments, even with some more acute cases.

Typically, appointments are two to three times per week, and we start off with approximately 12 visits, or four to six weeks. And depending on a person's progress, around that time we will reevaluate or do a progress exam to see how the patient is responding to the care. At this time, we may reduce the adjustment frequency to twice a week, eventually moving to once a week with the goal of spacing out the adjustments to once every two weeks after that.

Within that first month, I also give some home exercises to get the spine moving in between the chiropractic visits. That's the equivalent to brushing and flossing your teeth between your dental check-ups.

I will do more of the work in the beginning with the chiropractic adjustments, and then, with all the education we provide, we hand the torch over to the patients, so that they do more of the care at home and we do less of it in the office. Once our patients understand how to take care of their spine, the chiropractor's role is to provide a regular rhythm of maintenance care over a lifetime, as opposed to yo-yo-ing through constant recurring crisis care. It's important that patients become actively involved in getting better, and become pro-active about their health and recovery. Just as your dentist teaches you healthy dental habits to protect your teeth and gums, my role is to teach you what your spine needs to stay strong and healthy for your lifetime.

Points to Remember:

Typical chiropractic treatment consists of three phases: Evaluation, examination, and treatment. Each step is very important to achieve optimal results – reducing pain, while improving flexibility and range of motion. This protocol applies to people of all ages.

For chiropractic care to be successful, it is crucial to follow it on regular basis, or in other words, create a rhythm.

I hope you have found this chapter – and the other ones too, of course – interesting and informative. Next, I will explain what to do and not to do in order to improve your spinal health.

Stay tuned!

Chapter 5:
What It Will Take To Get Where You Want To Be

"Strength does not come from winning. Your struggles develop your strengths. When you go through hardships and decide not to surrender, that is strength."
- Arnold Schwarzenegger

"Focus on progress, not perfection."
- Dr. Mike

In the previous chapter, I outlined a typical chiropractic visit and treatment plan. I described what I, as a chiropractor, do to help reduce your pain, inflammation, and discomfort and move you towards full recovery with lasting results.

That is my role, and I take it very seriously. But you, the patient, as well as your extended network of family, friends, and colleagues, have an important part to play in your recovery as well. Let's look at the main components of your healing process.

Component #1: Family support

You are visiting a chiropractor to help you with low back pain (or whatever other problem brought you to my office). But while you start to feel much better, you still have weeks of treatment ahead of you. Can you count on the understanding and support of those closest to you?

I certainly hope so because various studies have shown that positive social support (from family, friends, and colleagues) plays a vital role in one's ability to manage limitations imposed by chronic pain.

Let me give you an example. In Chapter 1, I talked about my patient Mary, who suffered from chronic back pain. At times, her pain was so severe, she could hardly move. But Mary is lucky to have a supportive husband and teenage daughter. They not only encouraged her to get chiropractic care (sometimes even accompanying her to my office for the appointments) but they also made sure she did the exercises I recommended. "Sometimes I was just too tired to exercise," Mary told me, "but my daughter kept saying, 'Mom, you have to do this, it's for your own good.'"

Not surprisingly, Mary made good progress, and her rehabilitation and recovery went smoothly. To this day, she (and her family) takes the Omega-3, vitamin D, and probiotic supplements I recommended. They now all come in for regular spinal check-ups, and they feel and function great.

Now, imagine if Mary's husband and daughter were indifferent to her pain and did nothing to help her recover. Would she get better on her own? Probably, but the process could be slower and much more stressful. This principle applies to all health challenges and recovery, whether you have cancer, heart disease, or anything else that requires time: The support of your inner circle always helps with healing and recovery.

Component #2: Understanding The Healing Process

In order to make progress through your recovery, it is important to understand the three phases of healing.

In modern society, we have become used to thinking that most medical conditions can be cured with drugs – the "pop the pill and get better" mentality. This belief in "instant relief" and masking the symptoms does not work in harmony with nature and is not in alignment with the body's natural healing process. (This doesn't mean that there isn't a time and place for painkillers or emergency intervention).

Over the years, we have forgotten that in nature, healing takes time. There are some very specific biological phases that the body has to go through and these steps can't be skipped. You just can't fast-track them for the sake of convenience. The body will take its time to heal and the more you support it, the healthier and stronger your recovery will be.

In a moment, I'll outline the things that are beneficial to you during the recovery process. But for now, let's explore the topic of *healing* a little more.

As I already said, it takes time to get the spinal joints moving better and restore motion back into joints through the chiropractic adjustments. The first phase of healing is about 72 hours, during which the body might create a little bit of inflammation. It is a normal part of healing; that is when the surrounding blood vessels become a little bit leaky, releasing a lot of the healing factors and cofactors whose job it is to start the healing process. During this phase, some people may feel a bit achy, sore or sensitive.

The second phase is when the body lays down new tissues in the areas where the joints were kind of "rusty" and not moving well. And as we start to open up the joints and begin to restore proper motion, the body will create new tissues, very much like when a scar is formed on a wound.

In the beginning, this new tissue resembles a very unorganized pattern, which is laid down quickly to patch the area. This takes approximately four to six weeks. During this second phase of healing people will begin to feel a lot better. When that happens, a normal human reaction may be to say, "I am cured. I don't need any more treatment and I can stop my prescribed exercises!"

Actually, that's not the case. Feeling an improvement doesn't mean that the *entire* healing process is completed. The patch of restored tissues I just mentioned is not very strong yet, so stopping the treatment and exercises at this point is counterproductive and will not result in long-lasting benefits. But if patients continue beyond this point, they'll have a much lower risk of relapsing.

Component #3: Doing All the Right Things

As I noted above, family support is super important in the recovery process. But that doesn't mean you should rely exclusively on others to get better. The power over your health – both body and mind - is in *your* hands.

Here is a checklist of the things that pro-active patients should do during the healing process:

Move! The main thing that allows the body's tissues to become strong is *motion*. This is the third and final phase of the healing process. And it is the longest phase, potentially taking up to a year. Being sedentary has the opposite effect. Let's take the example of knee surgeries. Years ago, after the surgery doctors would put the leg in a cast and tell the patient: "Rest the knee. Don't move it!" That would be for the duration of the cast over several weeks. Afterwards, the knee was never the same – the tissues had not regained their strength or flexibility, and if you were a professional athlete your career was likely over.

Today, the understanding is totally different. As soon as the surgery is done, patients are put on a so-called motion machine to start the knee moving. This might have been a revelation to the medical community, but chiropractors have known all along that motion stimulates the body to strengthen the weakened tissues – be it in the knee or the spine. Nowadays it is common for high-end athletes to have knee surgery and come back to their sport "as good as new."

Spinal Hygiene! I don't mean soap and water; I am referring to exercise, which should be an integral part of any recovery program. Even though you may be tempted to lie down or take it easy, don't! It has been proven that exercise and motion help strengthen the spine, muscles, and joints, while improving range of motion and flexibility, and, ultimately, easing the pain.

Watching Your Weight! Being overweight is not only dangerous for your cardiovascular system and overall health, but it also puts pressure on your spine, knees, and joints in general. Carrying extra pounds actually hurts!

What can you do, and what are your options?

- You can follow a supervised and monitored keto-genic diet with a coach. This is designed to focus the body on burning fat, while preventing muscle loss. These one-on-one coaching programs are very easy to do and give people a satisfying, quick head start towards their health goals.

- You can follow a self-guided weight-loss program based on eliminating all grains, dairy, and processed sugars, all the while increasing your activity level.

- You can have a customized 90-day lifestyle plan made for you, which gives you everything you need to address physical, nutritional, and emotional aspects of health. This teaches you strategies on how to maintain your health for a lifetime.

Taking supplements! I can never sing enough praises to the importance of Omega-3, Vitamin D, and probiotics. I recommend these supplements to all my patients and have had excellent results. The science is absolutely clear: They aren't just a "good idea" or a fad or a temporary fix. They are essential for all humans. Our genetic code requires them to achieve health. All of us have a certain degree of deficiency in all these nutrients, so they are essential elements of the healing process – and beyond.

As a reminder, Omega-3 reduces inflammation (exactly what people who suffer from back and other pain need), and may also help lower the risk of chronic illnesses, including heart disease, cancer, diabetes, and arthritis. Vitamin D inhibits inflammation and is an integral part of the immune system response. And probiotics strengthen your body's immune system, improve digestion and aid in making B vitamins, among other healthy benefits. My patients see positive results of these supplements relatively quickly – certainly before all the healing phases mentioned above are completed.

Component #4: Staying The Course!

I said it before but I'll say it again: Lasting relief requires patience and perseverance! I already pointed out that there are three phases of healing – inflammation, regeneration, and remodeling - and it is crucial not to stop any of your care, (adjustments, home exercises and supplementation) as soon as the pain goes away.

Consistency is key! What we consistently do is what we consistently get! Flossing your teeth twice a year before you go to visit the dentist will never maintain the health of your gums and teeth the way flossing daily will.

I had a patient once, Jessica, who started to feel better after only two adjustments. She declared herself cured, and even though I attempted to explain to her the timeline and phases of healing, she had her own ideas and stopped all her care and "homework".

Obviously, I can't force my patients to continue the treatment against their will. When Jessica left, I had a feeling that I would be seeing her again, sooner rather than later. I was right: About a month later she came into the office and said her pain was back. I never tell patients "I told you so," because I understand that *experience* is often our greatest teacher. I am glad to report that the second time she was much more committed to completing her treatment and maintenance plan, and she has not had any relapses since!

Points to Remember:

It takes a committed and pro-active patient to get the most out of their chiropractic care. In the long run, this saves the person time, money, future pain, and potentially the loss of work time and enjoyment of life and hobbies.

During all the phases of healing, it is important to have the support and understanding of family and friends but, ultimately, it is up to the patient to follow all the steps towards better health: physical activity, exercise focused on regaining strength and mobility in the spine and joints, good eating habits, nutritional supplements, and tenacity.

In the next chapter, I will take the subject of results one step further: I will tell you how to get even more benefits out of your chiropractic care.

It just gets better and better!

Chapter 6:
How To Get Faster Results

*"Whether you are weeding the garden, taking care of your
teeth, or healing you spine, when you are an active participant
you will always get better results"*

In the previous chapter, I covered the process of results-driven recovery. It includes steps such as understanding the three phases of healing; doing exercises focused on regaining strength and mobility in the spine and joints; good eating habits and nutritional supplements; as well as being committed to treatment for as long as it takes to get lasting results (which can take up to a year).

Now I'd like to take this topic to the next level and talk about how you can be even more proactive in achieving spinal – and general – health.

Step #1: Prevention

You know the saying: An ounce of prevention is worth a pound of cure. This is as true of overall health as it is of your spine and joints.

Think of this car analogy: If you own a vehicle, chances are you keep it in good condition so it runs smoothly and safely. You don't want any of its vital parts to wear out and get rusty. What about your body? You certainly don't want it to wear out and get rusty because, while you can change the car's parts or get a new automobile, you only have one body.

Needless to say, you want to be really, really good to your body. And that means taking care of all of its parts and components.

One of the best ways to *prevent* (and not just treat) either chronic or acute pain is exercise. Yes, I know I have mentioned it before, but this point is so important, it merits repeating.

A recent study carried out at the University of Sydney and Macquarie University, both in Australia, and the Federal University of Minas Gerais in Brazil, found that "Exercise is the best medicine to banish back pain." These findings reiterate a number of earlier studies – as well as a lot of anecdotal evidence – showing that daily stretching and strengthening exercises (like the ones shown in the previous chapter) are the best way to keep back pain at bay.

But there is more to prevention than just exercise. Read on!

Step #2: Weight Loss

If you have been reading this book carefully, you know by now that overweight people have an increased risk for back and sciatica pain.

A recent patient of mine, Steven, carried most of his extra weight around the midsection, which caused his pelvis and abdomen to be pulled forward, creating stress on the lower back. No wonder Steven suffered not only from chronic lower back pain, but also from sciatica pain spreading down his right leg. Steven told me his doctor warned him that, unless he loses about 40 pounds, he could develop osteoarthritis – the degeneration of joint cartilage, the discs, and the underlying bone.

Steven was only in his mid-40s, so naturally he got scared and decided to get in shape. First, I adjusted his back, and then we sat down to discuss how he could lose weight safely. I told him about my weight and fat reduction program and he was eager to try it. Within a couple of months, Steven shed over 20 pounds and he is already feeling "lighter" – as he put it – and his pain has been greatly reduced.

He accomplished this with a diet, exercise, nutritional supplements (Omega-3, vitamin D, and probiotics), as well as regular adjustments in my office. Steven knows he is not out of the woods yet – he still has over 20 pounds to lose – but the positive result so far has given him motivation to stick to the program.

In Steven's case, the weight put pressure on his lower back – the lumbar spine. But I've had some patients whose excessive weight impacted many of their joints – knees and hips – causing irritation, pain and swelling. They too benefited from adjustments, along with the weight loss program and exercise.

The bottom line is this: the more weight you carry, the more wear, tear, and damage there will be on your spine and joints.

On the other hand, maintaining a healthy weight through diet and exercise not only alleviates existing pain, but also helps prevent these types of problems in the future.

Step # 3: Exercise

I know I have emphasized (and reemphasized) this point before, but I can't talk about good results without bringing up this subject again.

If you have ever had pain in your back or joints, chances are the last thing you wanted to do is exercise. But with the exception of extreme conditions (like fractures or disc herniations, for example), back exercises are not only recommended, but also actually *necessary* to rehabilitate the spine, help reduce the pain, stiffness, and weakness in muscles and ligaments. And, as I mentioned above, exercise will also prevent the recurrences of lower back pain or, in the very least, lessen the duration and severity of any future attacks.

Step #4: Stand Up and Get Moving!

It is probably no surprise that sedentary lifestyle not only leads to heart disease, diabetes, and several other serious conditions, but it also worsens back pain. That's because sitting for prolonged periods of time increases stiffness and weakens your muscles. It also stops you from being active and exercising – which, as I already mentioned, is essential for strong joints and spine.

My patient, Rebecca, is a good (or should I say "bad?") example of what can happen if you sit too much. Rebecca works from home and her job requires her to sit at her computer for many hours each day. Not surprisingly, when she came to see me, her discs already had early signs of degeneration and she was in pain. I treated her with a series of adjustments and she started to feel better. And although she promised to exercise more, she also told me that she could not change the "sitting" part of her day, since this was the only way she could do her work.

Things are as they are, and not always how we want them to be. In Rebecca's case, a complete overhaul of her lifestyle was not possible, so I suggested several small changes that would help lessen her pain and discomfort caused by all that sitting. For instance, I told her that correct sitting posture was very important – not to lean forward or slouch, as she had been doing (which can overstretch spinal ligaments), but, rather, to align her spine against the chair's back, keep her knees even with the hips, or a bit higher.

I also recommended that she take breaks from sitting every hour or so to get up, walk around, and stretch. I taught her appropriate spinal motion exercises that she can do throughout the day to counteract all the sitting she has been doing. She eventually started to work intermittently, standing at her kitchen counter, with her laptop raised up on a special portable laptop stand she purchased. Incidentally, the trend towards standing desks, or workstations is on the rise, due to the benefits of standing and the increased awareness of how harmful prolonged sitting is.

All throughout her initial care, her progress exams showed steady improvement. She continued to improve her flexibility, decrease her time sitting, and reduce the amount of inflammation in her body; also, she continually reports greater comfort in her day-to-day life.

Step #5: Avoid the "ouch" moments

Last year, Frank walked into my office. Actually, "walked" is an optimistic assessment of his posture. He *shuffled* in, bending at the waist, which is an all-too-common sight in a chiropractic office.

As it turned out, Frank was helping a friend move some heavy furniture and, as he explained, "something snapped in my back and I couldn't move." Upon examining him, I discovered that Frank irritated the joints in his lumbar spine and they were now "subluxated" - which is a fancy word for misaligned.

I helped Frank the best way I could – with gentle chiropractic adjustments to restore proper motion back into the lumbar joints - and he did feel some immediate relief. However, before I let him go, I explained how to safely lift heavy things – tips that anyone can use to avoid the kind of injury Frank sustained:

- Bend your knees, keep your back straight, and tighten your abdominal muscles.

- Keep your shoulders in line with your hips to avoid twisting.

- Hold the weight close to your body.

- Do not be a hero. Lift heavy objects with someone.

(Far too often in my career, I have seen patients whose spines were never the same after one heroic attempt to lift something they shouldn't have).

Step #6: Banish Stress

In a way, stress is like lower back pain: Nearly everyone experiences it. However, "life stress," sometimes referred to as emotional or mental stress – and anxiety that often goes with it – is detrimental to your overall health, including your spine.

That's because chronic mental stress or anxiety leads to increased muscle tension, which, in turn, increases pain – not just in your back, but also in the neck and shoulders. Stressful events increase the release of cortisol in the body, which has an inflammatory effect. Increased inflammation causes more tenderness and pain in the body. Perhaps you wouldn't think that stress can cause physical discomfort, but I have seen many patients in my practice whose sole source of pain seemed to be "life stress".

Joanna, for instance, told me that every time she became "tense or nervous," she could literally feel pain in her back and shoulders. I adjusted her, but also advised that she find an effective way to relax and de-stress, be it breathing techniques, yoga, meditation, or anything else.

And, I am sure it won't surprise you that I also recommended exercise. It produces endorphins — chemicals in the brain that act as natural painkillers – that help reduce stress and stress related aches.

If you follow all these guidelines and continue your chiropractic care for as long as needed, you will exponentially increase your chances of having strong and painless spine, joints, and muscles.

Now stay tuned because Chapter 7 is all about the life you can have and fun things you can do when you are pain-free.

Chapter 7:
What You Can Achieve When You Are *Not* In Pain

"Life shrinks or expands in proportion to one's courage."
- Anais Nin

Would you like to resume an activity you used to enjoy – or take up a new one you have always wanted to try –but your pain prevents you from doing so?

In this chapter, I will tell you what happens when you are not in pain –in other words, the advantages of being healthy and fit. Let's explore the three benefits of a pain-free life.

Benefit #1: Performance

Whether you work for a living, go to school, or are retired, you have certain tasks you need to do every day.

Whatever activity you're engaged in, your life is easier and much more pleasant when you're not in pain. That's the basic premise: When you're not in pain, you're happier.

There's a massive domino effect that happens when you're not suffering - everything from your performance and mood to how well you sleep. And when you sleep better, your immune system is much stronger, and the level of your inflammation goes down.

The domino effect doesn't stop there: When you are well rested, you focus better on whatever tasks you need to perform, and you enjoy your life so much more. You can try any kind of activities you want. You're not going to have pain holding you back.

The way I look at it is this: We may not all be super athletes in a sports arena, but we are all athletes in life.

Benefit #2: Sports

Most of us like some type of a sports activity – not necessarily at competitive levels, but simply for the pure enjoyment of it. Of course, you can only pursue this activity if your spine and joints are flexible and pain-free. It goes without saying that if you have a limited range of motion, there's no way you'll throw a ball very far, or do anything even slightly athletic.

A patient of mine, Greg, was an avid golfer. Now, golf is not necessarily an activity that requires the same kind of athletic skills as, say, hockey, but Greg's back and sciatica pain was so severe, he couldn't even turn, much less swing a club and hit a ball.

And another patient, Mark, had to temporarily abandon his weekly bowling game with his friends, because of his acute neck, shoulder, and arm pain.

Both Greg and Mark were extremely distressed that they had to give up their sports activities – something they had enjoyed for years. Besides the regular exercise and how it made their bodies feel, sports also provided some stress relief, allowed them to be connected with other people, and enjoy the social component of participating in an activity.

The good news is, that once I taught them the essential components of spinal health and how it is directly correlated to overall health, they both got better. I showed them how to improve, maintain and take care of their spines, and they both resumed their sports.

Benefit #3: Longevity and Quality of Life

Did you know that the human body is genetically designed for approximately 120 years of life? True, most of us will not reach that age, but that doesn't mean that we can't be active, vibrant, and energetic, no matter how old – or young – we are.

Many people don't realize that chronic pain can actually reduce their lifespan. How is this possible, you may ask? Well, the part of the brain that registers pain releases a number of hormones, including cortisol, the so-called stress hormone or the "fight or flight" hormone.

When released frequently over long periods of time, cortisol can have a detrimental impact on our health, leading to heart problems, high blood pressure, and the lowered capacity of the immune system.

All this is to say that when you are pain-free, the opposite happens: You can have a great quality of life and enjoy all your favorite activities.

So how do you get a pain-free life?

I have covered this topic in detail in previous chapters, but let's go over some important points again.

Point #1: Indulge Your Spine - Be Well Adjusted!

There are three categories of stress - the physical, chemical, and emotional.

In our modern world, it's very difficult to avoid these three types of stresses. They are ever-present in our lives. And as we are faced with those stresses, they continue to build up in our bodies, placing a tremendous load on the spine.

But when you get adjusted on a regular basis and keep the spine and joints moving properly, you don't allow that pressure to build up. This greatly reduces the chances of a crisis situation, when you suddenly are in acute severe pain.

I can tell you, based on my 20 years of chiropractic experience, that my patients who come in regularly every week or every two weeks to get adjusted, very rarely – if ever – find themselves in a crisis situation. That maintenance really pays off long term.

For instance, Debbie first came to see me five years ago, when she suffered from acute low back and sciatica pain. She was an avid biker but could no longer get on and off her bicycle – or use the pedals for that matter.

I gave her a series of adjustments, exercises to do at home, as well as Omega-3, vitamin D, and probiotic supplements. Debbie got progressively better and was eventually able to start biking again. This could have been the happy end of the story, but it wasn't.

To this day, Debbie comes to see me regularly every two weeks for adjustments. Not because she is in pain but because she *hasn't* been in pain since she started care five years ago!

On the other hand, I frequently see patients who have not continued their course of treatment for the recommended period of time. They started to feel better after a few adjustments and decided that was good enough.

You can probably guess what happened. Most of them come back to me after several weeks or months because the pain had returned. They tell me, "Doc, I should have listened to you and continued my treatment!"

This is not just my own experience: There are studies showing that only the patients who get regular, on-going care maintain their benefits and continue to improve.

So the science is clear. It shows that continued adjustments help keep the spine more flexible and functioning better, and mitigate the stresses that are building up in our day-to-day life.

And by the way, chiropractic care is not for adults only. I have many children in my practice, some of whom I've been adjusting since they were born.

Sometimes the birthing process can be quite rough on the baby's neck and spine, and so the adjustment protocol for an infant is very different from that used on adults: a very specifically focused light pressure with just the fingertips to assess where there may be some restrictions from the birthing process.

As kids grow and become more active, from learning to walk to starting new sports, they endure many bumps and falls, so it's very important to check their spine and pelvis regularly to make sure everything is as it should be. For healthy children, it's often enough to bring them in once every three to four weeks.

I've been treating many of the kids throughout most of their lives. When one of them, Zach, got to be 10 or 11, he started to play hockey. He fell and hurt himself plenty of times, and each time he'd tell his parents, "I got hit pretty hard today, I want to see Dr. Mike." Even without pain or an injury, kids start to learn early on in life that taking care of their spine preventatively will help them stay healthier and perform better. It is something they take with them as they get older and become responsible for their own health. Many of my adult patients went to a chiropractor regularly as children.

I am also adjusting a young girl. She is only 12, but has already developed quite a scoliosis. She has lived a long time with chronic back pain, until her mom started to bring her to me. Once we took care of the severe pain she was experiencing, she got on (and continues with) a regular schedule - once every three weeks. She is feeling and functioning so much better now, she is able to sit in class and compete in gymnastics without any pain or discomfort.

The protocol for adjusting kids is basically the same as for adults. The big difference is that children heal so much quicker and they bounce back faster than grown-ups. That's because the buildup of stresses hasn't yet happened to them, so an injury which would take up to three months to heal in an adult, might only require a two or three weeks of initial care treatment for a 10-year-old.

And, by the way, kids also require the Omega-3 and vitamin D supplements, but in smaller doses, based on their body weight. These essential nutrients are for all humans, not just adults.

Points to Remember:

When your spine and joints are pain-free and flexible, you can enjoy your life so much more. You become more efficient at your daily tasks – be it work, school, or any other activities; you are much better at sports; and your health and overall quality of life are boosted as well.

Regular – rather than sporadic – adjustments will give you all of the above benefits, and then some!

In the next chapter, I will expand on the subject I touched on before: Lifestyle, nutrition, and supplementation.

It's a fascinating topic, so keep on reading!

Chapter 8:
Lifestyle, Nutrition, and Supplementation

"The more you can choose foods that do not have an ingredients list, the better off you are. That means foods that come from the earth, unaltered. A general rule is that less processing equals a higher nutritional value."

As you know by now, I practice a holistic approach to health. Wellness is not simply a marketing word I use. In my office, wellness means that once people come to me, they will achieve higher levels of health.

In 20 years of practice I have seen the successes and the pitfalls my patients have experienced. I understand what it takes to achieve and maintain health. As much as chiropractic is the most effective, evidence-based care for spinal health, one has to address the person as a whole. When you add the right habits along with chiropractic care, the results become life changing!

Within that context, lifestyle, nutrition, and supplementation are very important for healthy and happy lives. Let's explore why.

Point #1: Lifestyle

I am going to repeat what I said before: Our lifestyle not only determines our health right now, but it also predicts how healthy, fit, and energetic we are likely to be in later years.

Basically, your overall current and future state of health is the outcome of either good or bad habits and behaviors, meaning: your lifestyle. Let's first look at the former –the positive and health-enhancing habits and behaviors in your daily life.

Number one is, of course, exercise, which is one of the main pillars of the healthy lifestyle, keeping your body and mind in shape and helping prevent many serious illnesses. Daily stretching and strengthening exercises also go a long way toward preventing spinal problems.

And if you already have back and, or joint pain, well-chosen exercises will rehabilitate the spine, and also help reduce pain, stiffness, and weakness in muscles and ligaments. Additionally, exercise will prevent the recurrences of lower back pain or, in the very least, lessen the duration and severity of any future attacks.

Another component of a healthy lifestyle – one that I talked about previously as well – is stress management.

Chronic stress and anxiety have been linked to medical conditions such as heart disease, cancer, stroke, depression, weight gain, and other serious illnesses. That's why lowering your stress level is so important to your overall physical and mental health.

There are different stress-reduction methods you could try, like breathing and relaxation techniques, meditation, yoga or massage. We are so lucky to have many professionals in our community who now teach yoga, others who give therapeutic and relaxation massages, and some very knowledgeable personal trainers who can ensure you are exercising safely and effectively.

Exercise has proven to be an effective stress-buster. In a previous chapter, I talked about endorphins, the body's chemicals in the brain that act as natural painkillers and help reduce stress and stress related aches. Exercise stimulates endorphin production, so you might say it's a natural "high." (And by the way, another thing that releases endorphins is laughter. It may not burn as many calories as exercise, but it will make you happy!)

Now that you know how to enhance your lifestyle, let's look at some things that you should definitely banish from your life:

- Sedentary lifestyle and inactivity – it promotes obesity, which, in turn, can lead to all kinds of illnesses including heart disease and diabetes. And all that sitting around is really, really bad for your spine because it weakens your muscles and causes stiffness.

- The extra pounds: Being overweight, as I mentioned earlier, puts a lot of pressure on the discs of your spine as well as on your knees, hips and feet. And, of course, it is detrimental to your cardiovascular and respiratory systems, and health in general.

- Smoking. Need I even list the reasons why cigarettes are bad for you? Let's see: Lung diseases (including cancer, emphysema and chronic bronchitis) heart disease, stroke, and a myriad of other health conditions. And I am not even mentioning aesthetic aspects like stained teeth and wrinkly skin. Thankfully smoking has been on a steady decline over the last couple of generations.

Okay, let's continue to explore things that have a *positive* impact on your health…

Point #2: Nutrition

You know the saying, "You are what you eat?" Well, it's true!

Unfortunately, far too many of us eat foods that are highly toxic to us – foods that are high in saturated fats, sodium, sugar, and various additives that not only wreak havoc with our weight, but also increase the risk of cardiovascular diseases, diabetes, cancer, and other serious illnesses.

Yes, I know, it's not always easy to eat healthy these days and get all the nutrients we need because so much of our food is processed and chemically treated (which is why we need good supplements; I'll talk about them in a minute).

There are some simple rules to good and healthy nutrition. They are not complicated, but if you are accustomed to the so-called "convenience" foods, or "fast foods," or any other kind of foods that may be pleasing to your palate but definitely detrimental to your body, you may need to adjust your eating habits quite a bit. But, believe me, in the end, it will be worth it!

So here are some of the guidelines:

- The more you can choose foods that do not have an ingredients list, the better off you are. That means foods that come from the earth, unaltered. A general rule is that less processing equals a higher nutritional value.

- The most impactful changes anyone can make are to reduce or completely eliminate carbohydrate intake from grains, dairy, and foods made with high-fructose corn syrup.

- Eat fresh, preferably organic and locally grown food, not industrial products. Generations ago food was just called food, until it became mass produced and chemically and genetically altered. For a few generations we never thought much about the chemicals being added to our food. Now the trend is reversing and we are seeing the availability of more and more organic food, which is bringing the costs down.

- With each meal, consume <u>raw</u> vegetables and, or fresh fruit. They are a great source of digestive enzymes, fiber, vitamins and minerals, water, and other nutrients.

- Drink lots of fresh, flat water. DON'T drink soda, either regular or diet.

- Season your food with only unrefined and unprocessed salt

- Cook with high-quality oils like olive, avocado or coconut, or butter from grass-fed cows. Avoid all hydrogenated oils and margarine, as they are chemically altered and toxic. The scientific community has made a complete reversal of its recommendations over the last 30 or so years, once telling us that fats were dangerous and causing heart disease and weight gain.

- The biggest culprit in the multitude of chronic illnesses from diabetes, cancer and heart disease is sugar, or anything that converts into sugar or glucose in our body after being digested. Glucose is what makes your fat cells expand and make you fat, and also feeds cancer cells, all the while suppressing your immune system and increasing inflammation.

- Talk to me about doing a sugar detox and find out what it can do for you. You'll be amazed at how good you feel!

The next question is: What foods should you consume on a regular basis? Here's a partial list:

- Grass-fed lean meat and free-range organic poultry.

- Wild-caught salmon.

- I know we are no longer used to eating organ meats, but if it comes from hormone and antibiotic-free, grass-fed animals, it is very healthy.

- Free-range organic eggs

- Organic, raw (not roasted) unsalted nuts and seeds.

- All the fresh fruits and vegetables you can, aiming for five servings of each per day.

If you need any more information about my nutrition plan, don't hesitate to contact me.

And if all of the above information is too overwhelming for you, remember that you don't have to change all your eating habits at once. Do it slowly, making one or two healthy choices every day, until it becomes an integral part of your life.

Just as the journey of a thousand miles begins with a single step, so does healthy nutrition start with just one spoonful!

Puppy Love 2

I'll retell this story as told by one of my mentors at one of the science of lifestyle seminars I attended:

Imagine at family at beautiful outdoor picnic. The picnic table is set and full of our traditional favourite picnic foods we all have grown to love. The little five year old girl in the family, reaches up into a large bowl on the table to grab a big handful of potato chips and she walks over to feed it to the family dog. The father notices this and quickly, just before the dog is about to eat the chips from her hand, yells out and grabs her arm to stop her. "No, no, honey!", he says to her, "we <u>never</u> feed the dog potato chips, that's <u>really bad</u> for him. No, honey, those chips are for <u>you</u>!"

I told you I had another funny dog story, only it's not that funny. We can see the absurdity of how many of us eat and think, how we treat ourselves and how we inherently know what is good for us.

Point #3: Supplements

If you eat a healthy and balanced diet, you probably don't need supplements; in fact, it's better not to take artificially synthesized vitamins in the multivitamin form. There is a concern that many of our foods, even the fresh raw veggies and fruit are not as nutrient-rich as they once were. The addition of a multivitamin made from fresh raw fruits and vegetables is the only kind of vitamin recommended. This type of product is not easy to find, but they do exist and I can recommend where to find one.

An alternate way of ingesting more vitamins and minerals is by juicing fresh fruits and vegetables. It doesn't replace your salad but is a great way to boost your nutrient intake.

There are a few ESSENTIAL nutrients that almost all of us are deficient in, no matter how well we eat, and those include: Omega-3 and vitamin D. And in addition to these two, I also strongly recommend a non-dairy based probiotic.

But let's begin with Omega-3. As I mentioned already, those of us living in western society are deficient in Omega-3. As we evolved over the millennia, we consumed a lot of this fatty acid in the natural environment in the form of wild game, organ meats, and the fish we ate.

With time, however, and certainly after the Industrial Revolution, our foods have changed dramatically. Farmers today feed the cattle corn rather than grass, and the meat has become very inflammatory. Remember what I said in a previous chapter: Our meat today is rich in Omega-6, which we need in equal amount to Omega-3. So while we get far more Omega-6 than we need, we have become deficient in Omega-3. Some research suggests that we now have 24 or 25 times more Omega-6 than we require.

This disproportionate ratio between Omega-6 and 3 produces an inflammatory response in the human body and so many of modern-day illnesses are caused by just that - inflammation. Anti-inflammatory drugs can never replace what your body lacks; all they do is artificially reduce the inflammation, instead of *treating* its cause, which is where Omega-3 can help.

The right quality and dosage is very important to pay attention to when supplementing with Omega 3s. Poor quality and / or too low of a daily dosage are the most common mistakes I find people make. You will end up wasting your money and, more importantly, your health will suffer. While Omega 3s are not a cure for anything, with a deficiency of Omega 3s your body can never be fully healthy. Thousands of research studies now support the important role Omega 3s play in our wellbeing.

One has to beware of what we read and what the source of the information is. It can be very confusing, even as a health professional. There is so much confusing information out there, and it's very easy to make a mistake by taking the wrong supplements, as I did early on in my life. If ever you come across articles that confuse you on the importance or the safety or the type of Omega 3 supplementation you need, come and talk to me. I can provide you with the science and the known quality brands that will help you.

Please make sure to get the proper advice on the brand and the dosage you are taking.

Now, let's move to vitamin D, which is created in our bodies through the exposure of UV-B light from the sun. Just like Omega-3, one of the things that happens in our body once we elevate our vitamin D levels, is that inflammation will be reduced, as well it also plays a large role in our immune defense against flus and cancer. Unfortunately, those of us living in North America – or anywhere in the world that's far from the equator - don't have enough of this vitamin.

Centuries ago, we got a lot of our vitamin D the same way we got Omega-3: through eating animal and organ meat because that's where a lot of the vitamins were stored. But since today we don't eat like that anymore, and we are told not expose ourselves to sunlight, the majority of us are dangerously deficient in vitamin D. As with any of the supplements I recommend, quality and dosage are important.

Last but not least are probiotics – these are the healthy bacteria in our gut, which is where our biggest defense mechanism and the greatest portion of our immune system live.

Eons ago, we used to get these healthy bacteria naturally from the food we consumed that came directly from the
earth. But since our food production methods and eating
habits have changed, we no longer get enough. In fact,
according to scientific literature, most of us are getting only
about one-millionth of the probiotics that we used to have
years ago.

There are also things that kill our healthy gut bacteria,
and one very common one is sugar. We are eating a lot of
it, much more than ever did and way more than we need.
Sugars can really damage the healthy bacteria in the digestive tract. Other things that are detrimental to the intestinal flora are antibiotics, artificial food coloring, increased
use of carbohydrates, certain medications (such as aspirin,
antacids, painkillers, and laxatives), and many other habits
and behaviors of the 21st century life.

These three supplements are the most scientifically
supported, yet deficient in most people. The addition of
Omega 3 and vitamin D to a chiropractic spinal care program creates much better outcomes for our patients. I love
doing progress exams on people who follow the protocol
exactly - they see and feel the results. This is often just
the beginning - they start adding more healthy habits and
reclaiming their lives!

As you already know, my practice is lifestyle oriented
and holistic, and I can't be holistic in the full sense of this
word, if I don't look at the whole person. Everything in the
human body is interconnected and interdependent.

These three supplements go a long way toward achieving wellness – both from the prevention and healing per-
spective. I'll be happy to provide more information, if you
wish. Feel free to contact me.

Points to Remember:

Healthy lifestyle and nutrition, along with supplementation, are very important for physical and mental wellness. Practicing these habits on daily basis will boost your general health and wellbeing, which extends far beyond just the spine.

In the next chapter, I will expand on this theme by exploring the importance and the extraordinary effects of a positive mindset for vitality, health and happiness.

This is one of my favorite subjects to talk about!

Chapter 9:
The Extraordinary Effect of a Positive Mindset for Vitality, Health and Happiness

"It's the repetition of affirmations that leads to belief. And once that belief becomes a deep conviction, things begin to happen."
- Muhammad Ali

There is a quote by Napoleon Hill that is very telling: "Whatever the mind can conceive and believe, it can achieve." This, in essence, summarizes the effect and the power of positive thinking.

Let's examine what impact a positive mindset can have on your health, vitality, happiness, and general wellbeing.

This is a truly fascinating subject!

In a way, it's all in your mind...

Unlike the brain, which is an actual organ, the mind doesn't exist in the physical sense. Yet, it enables us to have cognitive awareness, consciousness, thoughts, feelings, and perceptions.

For something that's not tangible, the mind holds tremendous powers. It determines how healthy, happy, and emotionally balanced we are. That's a big job for an organ that doesn't really exist!

The mind produces our thoughts, which, in turn, create feelings.

If we can master our thoughts, we'll also have the ability to master our emotions, behavior, and mental attitude.

So yes, it all really *is* in your mind!

Banish that thought!

People who have a negative mindset often suffer from various ailments. Why? Because the body responds to negative thoughts in a physiological and neurological way. For instance, it releases cortisol - the stress hormone I mentioned before – which increases the heart rate, blood pressure, glucose levels, and constricts blood vessels.

How many times have you thought of something disturbing, and immediately felt your heart pounding through your chest? Perhaps you also perspired a little bit, felt dizzy, had "butterflies" in your stomach, and other symptoms of anxiety? All that happened without you climbing a flight of stairs or doing any strenuous activity. You didn't do anything other than have a thought.

This is a good example of how our thoughts create changes in our physiology. And over time, we become accustomed to these chronic states of stress and, little by little, they damage our health, rob us of vitality, energy, and happiness.

As a matter of fact, scientific literature shows how negative emotions harm the body. For example, chronic stress or anxiety can alter biological systems, which, over time, cause "wear and tear" and, eventually, a slew of illnesses.

But it doesn't have to be this way.

Albert Einstein once said, "We cannot solve our problems with the same thinking we used when we created them."

He probably referred to physics, but this kind of thought process is very pertinent to our lives as well.

Basically, what this means is that if you have a negative mindset and live in a chronic state of stress and anxiety, all you'll be able to achieve are the symptoms I described above: The increased heart rate and blood pressure, and constricted blood vessels.

You are not solving any problems, but actually adding to and creating more.

True, some people are "naturally" more optimistic than others, so they have to work less at producing a positive mindset than others. But all of us can achieve this. Let's find out how.

Focusing on the bright side...

We all have the ability to choose our thoughts. One of the fairly simple ways to foster a positive mindset is to identify your core values of being a good person. That's a great place to start.

Core values are fairly universal, for example unconditional love for others and oneself. There are exercises we can do to identify our core values. Our values help us evaluate ourselves and others, and form our belief system. Our beliefs are what we use to assess our life experiences and help form our world.

As we know, our beliefs can change over time with different experiences and knowledge we acquire. Growing up in different parts of the world or in different families influences our beliefs. What we believe creates our internal dialogue.

We all have an internal dialogue that runs in the background every waking moment. Just like a muscle, that running dialogue is strengthened with repetitive practice. Once again, there are exercises one can do to become aware of our internal dialogue and change it, improving it over time.

The beauty of this is that it is not static or set in stone — it is under your control. Our beliefs influence our reactions. Our reactions may seem like a reflex far too ingrained to change, yet we all have power over our thoughts. Once we learn some strategies and practice them, we can drastically improve our outlook, thoughts, and reactions.

How we think, react, and what we believe can be shaped by our sense of gratitude or our practice of gratitude. Take this gratitude exercise below and see how often we might think the opposite of these statements:

Grateful for:

1. Early wakeups = Children to love

2. House to clean = Safe place to live

3. Laundry = Clothes to wear

4. Dishes to wash = Food to eat

5. Crumbs under the table = Family meals

6. Grocery shopping = Money to provide for us

7. Toilets to clean = Indoor plumbing

8. Lots of noise = People in my life

9. Endless questions about homework = Kids' brains growing

10. Sore and tired in bed = I'm still alive!

- Source unknown

I loved this example above, for it shows us just how easy it is to be grateful for the things so many of us complain about. I don't love any of those chores either, but it's a great reminder of how fortunate most of us are.

I constantly encounter and search for people who have a positive outlook, the kind of people who are seeking solutions rather than looking for problems. Remember: the types of people and news we expose ourselves to can shape our lives.

Let's go back to the example I cited before, the one about a negative thought releasing cortisol and causing unpleasant reactions in the body.

In this scenario, a scary or worrying thought starts to cause anxiety. You can either let it overpower you with palpitations, hyperventilation, sweating, etc.

Or, you can stay calm and think: "This is happening to me now. What can I do?"

First thing, take some deep breaths and focus on finding solutions to the problem that had just caused you such distress. That takes your mind away from the palpitations and hyperventilation, and channels it into a solution-oriented mode.

One of the things that science has shown us is that positive and empowering thoughts come from the left side of your brain. And through a complex series of pathways, those positive and empowering thoughts create nerve pathways that drive your body towards balance. And through similar series of pathways, the brain initiates a stress response in the body. So whatever pathway we repeatedly stimulate, the body will react to it more quickly and more easily.

Turning negative into positive

I once had a patient with Multiple Sclerosis and for many years she had to deal with a very abusive work environment. Obviously, this distressing situation caused her much anxiety and affected her overall health. She had very weak legs and arms and chronic tension headaches. She was tripping and falling, so she wasn't going for any walks. One of the biggest parts of her problem was that she had no hope. In her mind she was "doomed" and helpless. She had tried other avenues to deal with her health, but none offered any real hope and she always felt at the mercy of the healthcare provider.

After a thorough history and report of findings, I offered her some hope. Something she hadn't had in a long time. I gave her a plan for how she could help herself at home, and we put together a plan for getting her spine more mobile.

With a series of adjustments, I treated her pain and discomfort and, little by little, I saw her stress levels go down, her legs, arms and all the muscles getting stronger, and with her new outlook, her mood boosted.

When she saw all the improvements, self-esteem, confidence, and sense of empowerment replaced hopelessness and distress. She started to believe in herself and cut out some of the negative influences from her environment. Instead, she surrounded herself with positive people and positive influences, all of which started to help her train her "positive-thoughts-muscle". Like any aspect of health and life, what we repeat, with intention, or by habit, will start to grow.

We can't always change the world around us – in this patient's case, her work environment - but we can influence how we deal with life's adversities. And that's where a positive mindset makes all the difference! Every now and then I hear people make fun of positive thinking, and the use of positive affirmations. I remind them that every single one of us has self talk. So, it's your choice. You get to choose whether it's positive or negative self talk.

The benefits of positive thinking

So how does the positive mindset improve our health, happiness, and vitality?

As I already noted, positive outlook and attitude enable us to cope much better with stressful situations. And when we eliminate – or at least reduce – stress and distress from our lives, we also decrease the risk of high blood pressure, heart disease, obesity, stroke, diabetes, and many other illnesses.

And of course, the power of positive thinking also extends to our mental wellbeing. People who have positive thoughts are not as likely to be depressed as their negative-minded counterparts. They also have a better emotional balance and vitality, which foster a sense of enthusiasm and engagement (whereas negative / depressed people tend to be withdrawn).

The bottom line is this: Your mind is a powerful weapon. Depending on how you use it, it can either be your worst enemy or your best friend.

Points to remember:

Your mindset has a tremendous impact of how healthy and happy you are.

Positively minded people don't suffer as much from stress-related diseases as those with a pessimistic disposition. However, it is possible to change the pattern, turning negative thoughts into positive ones. Just like a muscle, the more we practice thinking positively, the more we practice gratitude, and the more it becomes our automatic default.

Do you have any questions about chiropractic? In the next chapter, which will be the last one of this book, I will answer many of the queries that my patients ask me. I hope my responses will provide all the information you may need.

Chapter 10:
Myths and FAQs*

"Great spirits have often encountered violent opposition from mediocre minds"
Albert Einstein

"90 percent of the stimulation and nutrients to the brain is generated by the movement of the spine."
-Dr. Roger Sperry,
Nobel Prize winner in brain research

I hope that in this book I have answered any questions you may have about chiropractic care in general and my practice in particular.

Just to cover all the bases, here are some typical questions I get. And since there are quite of few myths about what a chiropractor is and what he / she does, I am also addressing these misconceptions.

---

*   *The contents of this chapter is © Perfect Patients. Used with permission.*

FAQs

How does chiropractic work?

Chiropractic works because you are a self-healing, self-regulating organism controlled by your nervous system. Millions of instructions flow from your brain, down the spinal cord, and out to every organ and tissue. Signals sent back to the brain confirm if your body is working right. Improper motion or position of the moving bones of the spine called a "subluxation" can interfere with this vital exchange by irritating nerves and compromising the function of affected organs and tissues. Specific spinal adjustments can help improve mind/body communications. Health often returns with improved nervous system control of the body.

Do I have a slipped disc?

Between each pair of spinal bones is a disc. Its fibrous outer ring holds in a jelly-like material. This soft center serves as a "ball bearing" for joint movement. Because of the way a disc attaches to the spinal bones above and below it, it can't actually "slip". However, a disc can bulge. It can tear. It can herniate. It can thin. It can dry out. And it can collapse. But it can't slip.

Do I have a pinched nerve?

A pinched nerve is rare. It is more likely that an adjacent spinal bone irritates, stretches, rubs or chafes a nerve. These "subluxations" distort the nerve messages sent between the brain and the body. This can produce unhealthy alterations to the organs and tissues connected by the affected nerves.

How do you get subluxations?

There are three basic causes of subluxations. Physical causes could include slips and falls, accidents, repetitive motions and improper lifting. Emotions, such as grief, anger and fear can cause subluxations. Chemical causes could include alcohol, drugs, pollution and poor diet.

How do I know if I have a subluxation?

You can have subluxations and not even know it. Like the early stages of tooth decay or cancer, subluxations can be present before warning signs appear. The results of a thorough examination can show the location and severity of subluxations you may have.

Can subluxations clear up on their own?

Sometimes. Today's hectic lifestyles are a constant source of subluxations. Fortunately, our bodies have the ability to self-correct many of these problems as we bend and stretch, or when we sleep at night. When subluxations don't resolve, you need to see a chiropractic doctor!

What's an adjustment?

Chiropractic adjustments usually involve a quick thrust that helps add motion to spinal joints that aren't moving right. Some methods use the doctor's hands, an instrument, a special table, the force of gravity, or extremely light contacts. There are many ways to adjust the spine, each adapted to an individual's needs and comfort levels.

Are chiropractic adjustments safe?

Yes. A New Zealand government study found that adjustments are "remarkably safe". By avoiding drugs and risky surgery, chiropractic care enjoys an excellent track record. A thorough exam can identify the rare person for whom chiropractic care might be unsuited. Compare the statistics. Adjustments are safer than taking an over-the-counter pain reliever.

Will adjustments make my spine too loose?

No. Only the spinal joints that are "locked up" receive adjustments. This allows weakened muscles and ligaments to stabilize and heal.

Can the bone move too much?

Highly unlikely. A chiropractic adjustment is special. It has the right amount of energy, delivered to an exact spot, at a precise angle, at just the right time. The intent is to get a "stuck" spinal joint moving again, helping reduce nerve interference. Years of training, practice and experience make chiropractic adjustments specific and safe.

What makes the sound during the adjustment?

Lubricating fluids separate the bones of each spinal joint. Some adjusting methods can produce a sound when the gas and fluids in the joint shift. The sound is interesting, but isn't a guide to the quality or value of the adjustment.

Are all patients adjusted the same way?

No. Each patient's spine and care plan is unique. With 24 moving bones in the spine (that can each move in seven different directions!) we see a wide variety of spinal patterns. Each patient's care is custom tailored for his or her age, condition and health goals. You are unique and your care should be too.

Can I adjust myself?

No. Some people can make their joints "pop" but that's not an adjustment! Worse, damage can occur by mobilizing a joint with weakened muscles and ligaments. Adjustments are specific and take years to master. Even your chiropractic doctor must consult a colleague to benefit from chiropractic care.

How many adjustments will I need?

The number of adjustments varies with each patient and their individual health goals. Many patients sense progress within a week or two of frequent visits. Visits become less often as your spine stabilizes. In chronic cases, complete healing can take months or even years.

Why do newborns and children get adjustments?

Even today's "natural" childbirth methods can affect an infant's spine. Preliminary studies suggested that colic, unusual crying, poor appetite, ear infections or erratic sleeping habits can be signs of spinal distress. Pediatric adjustments are gentle. Knowing exactly where to adjust, the doctor applies no more pressure than you'd use to test the ripeness of a tomato.

Later, learning to walk, ride a bicycle, and other childhood activities can cause spinal problems. While a bandage and some comforting words can help a skinned knee, the unseen damage to the child's spine is the unique domain of a chiropractic doctor.

Many childhood health complaints that are brushed off as "growing pains" can often be traced to the spine. Regular chiropractic checkups can identify these problems and help avoid many of the health complaints seen later in adults.

Most parents report that their children enjoy their chiropractic adjustments and seem healthier than other children.

Am I Too Old For Chiropractic Care?

More and more people are consulting chiropractic doctors, especially in their later years. With growing concerns about over-medication and the side effects of combining various prescription drugs, safe, natural chiropractic care is growing in popularity.

Restoring better spinal function can help improve mobility, vitality, endurance, and appetite. Many patients report improvements with arthritic symptoms and other chronic ailments often falsely attributed to aging. Your chiropractor will modify their adjusting technique for maximum comfort and results.

Can I have chiropractic care after back surgery?

Yes. Rest assured that your chiropractic doctor will avoid the surgically modified areas of your spine. Surgery often causes instability above or below the involved level. These areas will be the focus of your chiropractic care.

Can patients with osteoporosis get chiropractic care?

Of course. When developing a care plan, your chiropractic doctor considers the unique circumstances of each patient. There are many ways to adjust the spine. The method selected will be best suited to your age, size and health.

How long until I'll feel better?

Some patients experience almost instant relief. Others discover it can take many weeks or months. Many factors can affect the healing process. How long have you had your problem? Are you keeping your appointments? Are you getting the proper rest, exercise and nutrition? Do you smoke? Are you in otherwise good condition? Within a short period of time most patients sense enough progress to fully complete their doctor's recommendations.

How long will I need chiropractic care?

After patients get the relief they want, many choose to continue with some type of periodic care. These patients show up for their visits feeling great. These visits can help support the final stages of healing and help detect and re-solve new problems before they become serious. Our job is to offer the very best care and your job is to decide how much of it you want.

Will I receive any medication for my pain?

No. Chiropractic doctors don't dispense drugs. Because we rely on natural methods, we can show you how to use ice to control painful symptoms. When properly applied, ice can have an analgesic effect without the side effects of pain medications.

Why don't medical practitioners and chiropractic doctors get along?

That's changing. Years of prejudice and bias are giving way to research showing the benefits of chiropractic care. Attitudes are slow to change. However, as the public de-mands alternatives to drugs and surgery, more and more medical practitioners are referring their patients to chiro-practors. Many chiropractors enjoy good relations with lo-cal doctors, to their patients' benefit.

What if my policy doesn't cover chiropractic?

Your health affects everything you do and everyone you know. It is your most valuable possession. Yet, each of us is free to place a different value on our health. It's convenient when an insurance company or third party helps pay the bill. But be careful! Don't allow the profit motive of a huge corporation to make the decision for you.

Will I ever be normal again?

Patient results vary. Many report improved spinal curves and the total resumption of their life. Those who have neglected or delayed seeking care often see slower progress. After improvement, many patients discover that periodic chiropractic checkups can help avoid a relapse.

What if chiropractic doesn't work?

If we're unable to find and correct the cause of your particular health problem, we will refer to other specialists who may be able to help. Your health is our only goal.

Busting the myths

If you have doubts, join the club. Chiropractic is different. And it is this difference that has brought results to millions and caused them to rethink the nature of health and the role of chiropractic care in it.

Once and for all, let's put to rest some of the most common myths:

Myth #1: Chiropractic isn't scientific

If you define it as the systematic pursuit of knowledge involving the recognition of a problem, the collection of data through observation and experiment and then testing the resulting hypotheses, then today's chiropractic is quite scientific. Because it's based on the scientific fact that the nervous system controls and regulates virtually every cell, tissue, organ and system of the body.

Don't be misled by the "low-tech" nature of chiropractic adjustments! There are a growing number of studies that suggest the chiropractic approach to reducing nerve disturbance along the spine, may enhance the ability of the brain and nerve system to control and regulate the body.

These include published research documenting the results of chiropractic care on asthma, infantile colic, immune function, dysmenorrhea (menstrual cramps), improving vision and brain function, lower back pain, one's overall health status and many others.

The "scientific" argument is largely a red herring and the sign of a double standard. Medical economist David Eddy, MD, Ph.D., observes that only 15% of medical procedures have ever been scientifically verified, and the other 85% of common medical procedures have no "scientific basis!"

Ultimately, the proof is in the pudding. Ask our delighted patients whether chiropractic is scientific.

Myth #2: Chiropractors are poorly educated

The fact is, educational requirements for today's chiropractor are among the most stringent of any of the health care professions.

Several decades ago the education that chiropractors received was purposely narrow. Without the interest in prescribing medicines or performing surgery, chiropractic education focused on anatomy, the philosophy of natural healing, the wisdom of the body and adjusting techniques.

Today's chiropractor receives a much broader education. In fact, it's quite comparable to that received by medical practitioners. Before acceptance to a five-year chiropractic college, prospective chiropractors must complete a minimum of three years of undergraduate work with a heavy emphasis on the basic sciences.

This focus on science continues during the first two years of study, emphasizing classroom and laboratory work in anatomy, physiology, public health, microbiology, pathology and biochemistry. Later, the focus is on specialized subjects, including chiropractic philosophy and practice, along with chiropractic diagnosis and adjusting methods. Since chiropractors don't prescribe drugs, instead of studying pharmacology and surgery, they receive an even deeper training in anatomy, physiology, rehabilitation, nutrition, diagnosis, X-ray and a variety of adjusting techniques that aren't taught in any other health care field.

Disparaging the educational achievements of today's chiropractor is an outdated belief from another era.

Myth #3 Chiropractors aren't real doctors

Your notion of a "real" doctor probably conforms to a prototype generated by the mass media.

Many have come to think of a doctor as someone who prescribes advice and drugs or performs surgery. Sporting a white lab coat or surgical scrubs with a stethoscope at the neck, doctors are seen as all-knowing, omnipotent and able to save patients in 60 minutes, less commercials.

A medical doctor (MD) and a chiropractor (DC) - while different - have both received a degree from a government accredited medical school or chiropractic college and are licensed to practice.

But that's where the similarity ends because each discipline looks at health and healing in very different ways.

Myth #4: Chiropractic adjustments cause stroke

The argument about safety concerns is an example of "junk science" and a perennial favorite by those who have an interest in discouraging people from seeking chiropractic care.

Because of the popularity of this tactic, year after year it has been the subject of countless research projects. The result of these studies shows complications from neck adjustments, the supposedly "riskiest" chiropractic procedure, are exceedingly rare:

1972 – One death in several tens of million adjustments.
1978 – One in 10,000,000 neck adjustments.
1981 – One in a 1,000,000 neck adjustments.
1983 – Two to three per 1,000,000 adjustments.
1985 – One in 400,000 neck adjustments.
1993 – One in 3,846,153 neck adjustments.
1995 – One in 2,000,000 neck adjustments.
1996 – One in 900,000 neck adjustments.

The most recent in-depth review of the relationship between stroke and chiropractic care, was published in the February 15, 2008 issue of Spine Journal. It looked at 10 years of hospital records, involving 100 million person-years.

The verdict?

There was no evidence of an increase in vertebral artery dissection risk with chiropractic, compared with medical management. Based on this review, stroke, particularly vertebrobasilar dissection, should be considered a random and unpredictable complication of any neck movement, including cervical manipulation.

In other words, cases of serious injury are practically

nonexistent. By comparison, it makes the deaths caused by over-the-counter-pain-relievers to be considerably more troubling! Although reports vary, annual deaths in the United States attributable to NSAIDs (Non-Steroidal Anti-Inflammatory Drugs such as aspirin, ibuprofen, naproxen, diclofenac, ketoprofen and tiaprofenic acid) range from 3,200 to higher than 16,500 deaths and 76,000 hospitalizations.

Even risk-averse insurance companies recognize the safety of today's chiropractic care. The premiums for malpractice insurance paid by chiropractors are a mere fraction of what medical practitioners must pay. Chiropractic care is safe.

Myth #5: Once you go, you have to go for the rest of your life

We've all heard the joke, "How many chiropractors does it take to change a light bulb?

Only one but it takes 100 visits."

Funny. Ha-ha.

The fact is, you don't have to do anything you don't want to. Many folks choose to continue their chiropractic care on some type of periodic basis for the rest of their lives.

Others choose to see us from time to time for episodes of neck or back pain. It's your choice. However, this concern is prompted by two common questions:

"Will I get addicted to chiropractic adjustments?"

No. Many people feel a pleasant sense of ease and well-being after their chiropractic adjustments. Some feel as though their power has been "turned on."

Others feel more whole or "connected." (This is what "normal" feels like!) Once people experience this feeling they often choose to adopt some type of ongoing schedule of care so they continue to feel this way all the time. It's not an addiction.

"Why are so many visits necessary?"

By the time many people consult our practice, they've had their problem for some time. Retraining muscles and ligaments that support the spine takes time. Each visit builds on the ones before. Remember, you're doing the healing, not the chiropractor!

How long you decide to benefit from chiropractic care is always up to you.

Myth #6: Don't fix it if it isn't broken

This is the "Let sleeping dogs lie" approach to health care! I feel fine. Why do I need to see a doctor?

That's the problem with the lifestyle-induced health problems facing our culture. They quietly fester in the background, slowly worsening, often without any obvious symptom. Arterial plaque builds up. Blood pressure rises. Certain foods now cause heartburn. Every morning you get out of bed a little bit slower and stiffer. You hardly notice the incremental change.

Ironically, these are often the same folks who religiously change their oil and do other preventive maintenance to lengthen the life, appearance and performance of their car!

If you like being your very best, you'll love visiting our practice. No shots. No yucky medicine. No "healthier-than-thou" attitude. No preaching.

Myth #7: My medical doctor wouldn't approve

Most medical doctors are unfamiliar with chiropractic and the principles by which it works. Many are still operating under the policy perpetuated by the illegal boycott of chiropractors by the American Medical Association in the United States and the Australian Medical Association in Australia.

On September 25, 1987, a United States Federal judge ruled that the AMA had violated Section 1 of the Sherman Act, and that it had engaged in an unlawful conspiracy in restraint of trade "to contain and eliminate the chiropractic profession." The judge issued a permanent injunction against the AMA under Section 16 of the Clayton Act to prevent such future behavior.

Fortunately, more and more enlightened medical doctors around the world see the value in chiropractic care.

"Instead of thinking of chiropractic as an alternative or some kind of therapy separate from other health care, we really should consider it equivalent."
Paul Shekelle, M.D., Ph.D.
The RAND Corporation

Myth #8: Chiropractic isn't appropriate for children

Why would a child have a spine and nervous system problem? Traumatic births. Learning to walk. Slips. Falls. The list is endless. Yet, because children have such an adaptive capacity, these problems are often brushed off as "growing pains" or just a "phase they're going through."

"As the twig is bent, so grows the tree."

Many patients report that chiropractic care has been helpful for colic, ear infections, erratic sleeping habits, bed wetting, scoliosis, "growing pains" and many other common childhood health complaints.

The concern that many parents have is that chiropractic adjustments will be too forceful. They mistakenly think that their child will receive adjustments like ones they receive. Not only are adjusting techniques modified for each person's size and unique spinal problem, an infant's spine rarely has the long-standing muscle tightness seen in adults. This makes a child's chiropractic adjustments gentle.

Knowing exactly where to adjust, newborns and infants are adjusted with no more pressure than you'd use to test the ripeness of a tomato. Many parents have commented that they see almost instant improvements in the well-being of their child.

Myth #9: You need a referral to see a chiropractor

You don't need a referral or permission from anyone to see a chiropractor.

However, if you expect financial assistance from certain insurance plans, some policies dictate that certain approval steps be taken before commencing care. Sometimes these are granted freely and sometimes it's virtually impossible.

Be careful that you don't allow your health to be compromised by the profit motives of an insurance company or the petty bias or jealousy of a gatekeeper who doesn't understand chiropractic!

It's your body, your health and your future.

Myth #10: Chiropractic results are just placebo effect

Some dismiss the results our practice members receive as merely the placebo effect. These cynics virtually ignore the mind/body connection that most forward-thinking health care experts are finally acknowledging.

A placebo (from the Latin 'I will please') is often a sugar pill or some type of sham treatment designed to invoke the beliefs of the patient, and in the case of double blind studies, even the beliefs of the doctor. Some studies show that placebos can be 30% to 40% effective.

Should the consistent results that today's chiropractic

practice member enjoys be simply chalked up to the place-bo effect and a caring personality?

Hardly. While it's helpful when the patient believes the care they're receiving will help them, some chiropractors have seen positive results from helping newborns, infants and even animals for which the power of the believing mind is clearly not a factor.

Conclusion

"Simplicity is the ultimate sophistication"
-Leonardo Da Vinci

We are what we repeatedly do.
Excellence, then, is not an act, but a habit."
- Aristotle

I t is so important to keep things simple and get back to the basics of health, so that you can spend time doing what you love and living life on your own terms. That's why I have an easy lifestyle questionnaire that you can do from home that will show you where you are today and what steps to take to heal, strengthen or protect your health, all depending on your starting point.

A lot of people are so confused with all the trends, fads and marketing, that they have trouble figuring out where to start, what to do and what <u>not</u> to do. They waste precious time, going in circles, or, they just avoid the whole subject because it seems too difficult. When we use the laws of biology and nature to guide us, it becomes very easy to see why and how we are getting sick and how simple it is to create health.

Most of the time, when people come to see me, it's because of some nagging pain or a major crisis.   Some people will already have a home routine, maybe a diet, or exercises or supplements they are taking to improve their health or lose a few pounds. Sadly, many of the things I hear on my first consult are the wrong approach and will never give them the results they want. It becomes so costly for people to waste their time doing the wrong things, following the latest fads or wrong advice, and their decline in health starts affecting the ability to do their job, being active in family life, affecting relationships, moods and overall quality of life.

Since the spine is at the core of your body, and it affects all aspects of your life, that will almost always be what I assess first.   Like a first check-up for your teeth and gums, I'll see where you are and find out what needs to be done.

I will help you identify your current status; find out what's causing the problem; tell you the solutions for healthy recovery, and then, what steps you can take for prevention and to make you feel and look young again.

For those of you who are not currently in a crisis, but want to find out where you are for your age, if you are on the right track and where you are headed, you can go to my website: www.AdioChiro.ca or call (613) 443-3511 and request a free 15 minute consult to come in and discuss your current status and your goals with me and figure out the perfect direction for you to take. When you book your appointment online or by phone, simply use the code Wellness 123 Free 15.   In that time we can discover what is the most important first step for you. This will also give you access to a full spinal and health assessment.

I'm excited that you are taking steps to a greater and

healthier you, and I am here to guide and show you how you can become independent and in control of your health. I know the impact it will have on your life, career, family and your overall happiness will be transformative.

I wish you great success and health freedom, all while keeping it simple.

Dr. Mike

About Dr. Mike and
ADIO Family Chiropractic

Dr. Michael Koschade is solutions oriented, using science-based wellness to focus on client's individual goals, using referenced facts, measurable results and ultimately showing people how they can achieve health freedom.

His specialty is making health easy to understand, keeping it simple and ensuring that people get on the right track. He helps clients focus their time and effort on the things that will give them the greatest results and have the biggest impact on their enjoyment of life.

Products and Service Offerings

1. Crisis Pain Care.

We help you get moving and out of pain as efficiently and effectively as possible. We will not simply cover up your symptoms, we'll determine the cause or causes are. We'll assess your problem, note your abilities and limits, take x-rays if needed, and create a report for you which outlines where you are and what you need to do to get out of pain and heal your body.

The system we use measures your progress along the way so that you can see and feel how you are improving. We use the latest sciences to determine where you are for your age and what you need to get better.   As we work together to get you out of your crisis situation, we'll also figure out how and what caused the problem in the first place and what you need to do to avoid this in the future.

2.   Chronic Recurrent Problem Care

So many people live with pain they think is "normal". Pain is there, for one reason and one reason only, to tell us to "pay attention". Pain is a signal to the brain to tell us to modify our behavior in a way to stop creating harm and allow the body to heal.   For those people who have an ongoing, repetitive problem, that may come and go, or may always be there, perhaps it's gradually getting worse over the years, but have learned to "live with it", the same process applies. We will determine where you are, and assess what is causing the problem.   Once we know what the cause is we can determine what is needed to fix the problem.

3.   Wellness / Performance Care

For those who feel well and healthy yet are interested in making sure they are on track, and, or, want the best advantage for a long healthy life.   For those who have never had a spinal check-up, or did years ago and know it's time to get checked again. Like a dental check-up, along with proper, regular maintenance habits, your spine can serve you very well for a lifetime with proper regular care.

4. One-on-One Weight-loss Coaching

For those who want to lose weight and have tried on their own, we provide an easy to follow medically-based approach. We provide the education and understanding of how the human body uses and stores energy as fat. We'll highlight the most common pitfalls and why working out and eating less doesn't get the results that are wanted or needed. We'll also show clients how to be successful in maintaining their results once they've achieved their goals. We meet with our clients weekly to take measurements and ensure they are maintaining their muscle mass and are staying on the right track.

5. 90 Day Lifestyle Plans

This is for the person who wants to address their lifestyle as a whole. How they eat, how they move and how they think. It is a complete above-down, inside-out, step-by-step process covering 90 days of food, exercise and thought patterns. It is a powerful tool to learn how to become self sufficient and in control of all areas of life.

To take advantage of any of these services,
or to find out more information,
please contact us at
www.AdioChiro.ca or call (613) 443-3511